Official Journal of the

European Association of Urology

EORTC
European Organization for Research and Treatment of Cancer – Genito-Urinary Group

ESUOE
European Society for Urological Oncology and Endocrinology

European Urology

KARGER

Printed in Switzerland on acid-free paper by Druckerei Schüler AG, Biel

Appears monthly: 2 volumes per year (12 issues)

Guidelines for Authors

European Urology

Submission

Only original papers written in English are considered and should be sent to:

Prof. C.C. Schulman
c/o S. Karger AG
Editorial Department of European Urology
PO Box
CH–4009 Basel (Switzerland)

Manuscripts should be submitted in triplicate (with three sets of illustrations of which one is an original), typewritten double-spaced on one side of the paper, with a wide margin.

Conditions

All manuscripts are subject to editorial review. Manuscripts are received with the explicit understanding that they are not under simultaneous consideration by any other publication. Submission of an article for publication implies the transfer of the copyright from the author to the publisher upon acceptance. Accepted papers become the permanent property of 'European Urology' and may not be reproduced by any means, in whole or in part, without the written consent of the publisher. It is the author's responsibility to obtain permission to reproduce illustrations, tables, etc. from other publications.

Arrangement

Title page: The first page of each paper should indicate the title (main title underlined), the authors' names, and the institute where the work was conducted. A short title for use as running head as well as the full address of the author to whom correspondence should be sent are also required.

Full address: The exact postal address complete with postal code must be given at the bottom of the title page. Please also supply phone and fax numbers, as well as your e-mail address.

Key words: For indexing purposes, a list of 3–10 key words in English is essential.

Abstract: Each paper needs an abstract of up to 16 lines structured with subheadings as follows: Objective(s), Methods, Results, Conclusion(s).

Small type: Paragraphs which can or must be set in smaller type (case histories, test methods, etc.) should be indicated with a 'p' (petit) in the margin on the left-hand side.

Footnotes: Avoid footnotes. When essential, they are numbered consecutively and typed at the foot of the appropriate page.

Tables and illustrations: Tables and illustrations (both numbered in Arabic numerals) should be prepared on separate sheets. Tables require a heading and figures a legend, also prepared on a separate sheet. For the reproduction of illustrations, only good drawings and original photographs can be accepted; negatives or photocopies cannot be used. Due to technical reasons, figures with a screen background should not be submitted. When possible, group several illustrations on one block for reproduction (max. size 181 × 223 mm) or provide crop marks. On the back of each illustration, indicate its number, the author's name, and 'top' with a soft pencil.

Color illustrations: Up to 6 color illustrations per page can be integrated with the text at the reduced price of CHF 660.– / USD 545.00 per page. Color illustrations are reproduced at the author's expense.

References: In the text identify references by Arabic numerals [in square brackets]. Material submitted for publication but not yet accepted should be noted as 'unpublished data' and not be included in the reference list. The list of references should include only those publications which are cited in the text. Do not alphabetize; number references in the order in which they are first mentioned in the text. The surnames of the authors followed by initials should be given. There should be no punctuation other than a comma to separate the authors. Cite all authors, 'et al' is not sufficient. Abbreviate journal names according to the Index Medicus system. (Also see International Committee of Medical Journal Editors: Uniform requirements for manuscripts submitted to biomedical journals. Br Med J 1988;296:401–405.)

Examples

(a) Papers published in periodicals: Sun J, Koto H, Chung KF: Interaction of ozone and allergen challenges on bronchial responsiveness and inflammation in sensitised guinea pigs. Int Arch Allergy Immunol 1997;112:191–195.

(b) Monographs: Matthews DE, Farewell VT: Using and Understanding Medical Statistics, ed 3, revised. Basel, Karger, 1996.

(c) Edited books: Parren PWHI, Burton DR: Antibodies against HIV-1 from phage display libraries: Mapping of an immune response and progress towards antiviral immunotherapy; in Capra JD (ed): Antibody Engineering. Chem Immunol. Basel, Karger, 1997, vol 65, pp 18–56.

Further details: Authors may consult our leaflet 'Rules for the Preparation of Manuscripts', available on request from the Publisher, S. Karger AG, P.O. Box, CH–4009 Basel (Switzerland).

Rapid Communication: Manuscripts intended for rapid communication must present new findings of sufficient importance to justify their accelerated acceptance. They should follow the general arrangement of research papers with the exception that no abstract or introduction are required. The first paragraph should include the reason for the study and the main findings. They should not exceed 8 double-spaced manuscript pages in length, including figures, tables and references. Proofs are checked by the Main Editor and not sent to the author. Review will be rapid, and once accepted, the paper will be included in the next planned issue.

Galley proofs

Unless indicated otherwise, galley proofs are sent to the first-named author and should be returned with the least possible delay. Alterations made in galley proofs, other than the correction of printer's errors, are charged to the author. No page proofs are supplied.

Reprints

Order forms and a price list are sent with the galley proofs. Orders submitted after the issue is printed are subject to considerably higher prices. Allow five weeks from date of publication for delivery of reprints.

KARGER

Fax +41 61 306 12 34
E-Mail karger@karger.ch
www.karger.com

The Guidelines for Authors are available at:
www.karger.com/journals/eur/eurinst.htm

General Information

European Urology

Publication data: 'European Urology' is published 12 times annually. Volumes 33–34 with 6 issues each appear in 1998.

Subscription rates: Subscriptions run for a full calendar year. Prices are given per volume.

Personal subscription:
Subscription + postage and handling
CHF 332.– + CHF 23.50 Europe
CHF 332.– + CHF 35.50 Overseas
USD 241.20 + USD 23.50
(Must be in the name of, billed to, and paid by an individual. Order must be marked 'personal subscription'.)

Institutional subscription:
Subscription + postage and handling
CHF 664.– + CHF 29.40 Europe
CHF 664.– + CHF 44.40 Overseas
USD 522.00 + USD 29.40

Airmail postage: CHF 24.–, USD 20.00.
(Extra per volume.)

Discount subscription prices:
European Association of Urology
European Organization for Research and Treatment of Cancer – Genito-Urinary Group
European Society for Urological Oncology and Endocrinology

Microforms: Please direct all enquiries and orders to: University Microfilms Inc.
300 North Zeeb Road, P.O. Box 1346
Ann Arbor, MI 48106-1346 (USA)

Subscription orders: Orders can be placed at agencies, bookstores, directly with the Publisher
S. Karger AG, P.O. Box,
CH–4009 Basel (Switzerland)
or with any of the following distributors:
Deutschland: S. Karger GmbH, Postfach
D–79095 Freiburg
France: Librairie Luginbühl
36, bd de Latour-Maubourg, F–75007 Paris
Great Britain, Ireland: S. Karger Publishers
58 Grove Hill Road
Tunbridge Wells, Kent TN1 1SP
USA: S. Karger Publishers, Inc.
26 West Avon Road, P.O. Box 529
Farmington, CT 06085
India, Bangladesh, Sri Lanka:
S. Karger India Subscription Agency
B–5/132 Safdarjung Enclave
New Delhi-110029
Japan: Katakura Libri, Inc.
Take 1 Bldg, 2nd Floor, 4-5-7 Yushima
Bunkyo-ku, Tokyo 113

Change of address: Both old and new address should be sent to the subscription source.

Single issues and back volumes: Information can be obtained through the Publisher.

Advertising: Correspondence and rate requests should be addressed to the Publisher.

Bibliographic indices: This journal is regularly listed in bibliographic services, including *Current Contents®*.

KARGER

Fax + 41 61 306 12 34
E-Mail karger@karger.ch
www.karger.com

The Journal Home Page is available at:
www.karger.com/journals/eur

Urinary Tract Cancer: State of the Art

EORTC GU Group Seminar

Editor: Louis Denis

This supplement issue presents advances in knowledge of the main urological cancers from a multidisciplinary perspective. It opens with an in-depth overview of controversial issues in the diagnosis and treatment of prostate cancer, followed by a paper on animal models and preliminary experience with oral bropirimine in phase I–II trials. The next four presentations focus on superficial bladder cancer, and include an overview of recent literature and results from ongoing clinical trials. Further contributions demonstrate the importance of randomized clinical trials to the care of patients with bladder cancer and provide a complete review of the diagnosis and treatment of kidney cancer. The final papers deal with important, but often ignored, subjects: quality of life, statistical design of trials and health economics. Bringing together the expertise and experience of leading authorities, this issue is valuable reading for all those interested in optimizing the treatment of patients with urinary tract cancer.

Contents

European Urology
Editor: Schulman, C.C. (Brussels)
ISSN 0302–2838
Supplement issue: Vol. 31, Suppl. 1 (1997)
Included in subscription

Urinary Tract Cancer: State of the Art
EORTC GU Group Seminar
Editor: Denis, L. (Antwerp)
VI + 82 p., 27 fig., 17 tab., soft cover, 1997
CHF 80.– / DEM 96.– / USD 69.75
Prices subject to change
DEM price for Germany, USD price for USA only
ISBN 3–8055–6466–X

Fields of Interest: Urology; Oncology; Chemotherapy

KI 97629

KARGER

European
Urology

Uroselectivity: Myth or Reality?

Satellite Symposium
held during the IVth International
Consultation on BPH
Paris, France, July 2–5, 1997

Guest Editors
Karl-Erik Andersson, Lund
Roger S. Kirby, London

11 figures, and 17 tables, 1998

KARGER
Basel · Freiburg · Paris · London · New York ·
New Delhi · Bangkok · Singapore · Tokyo · Sydney

KARGER

S. Karger
Medical and Scientific Publishers
Basel · Freiburg · Paris · London
New York · New Delhi · Bangkok
Singapore · Tokyo · Sydney

Drug Dosage
The authors and the publisher have exerted every effort to ensure that drug selection and dosage set forth in this text are in accord with current recommendations and practice at the time of publication. However, in view of ongoing research, changes in government regulations, and the constant flow of information relating to drug therapy and drug reactions, the reader is urged to check the package insert for each drug for any change in indications and dosage and for added warnings and precautions. This is particularly important when the recommended agent is a new and/or infrequently employed drug.

P.O. Box, CH–4009 Basel (Switzerland)
Printed in Switzerland on acid-free paper by
Druckerei Schüler AG, Biel
ISBN 3–8055–6550–6

Contents Vol. 33, Suppl. 2, 1998

European Urology

KARGER

Fax+ 41 61 306 12 34
E-Mail karger@karger.ch
www.karger.com

Access to full text and tables of contents,
including tentative ones for forthcoming issues:
www.karger.com/journals/eur/eurcont.htm

European
Urology

Introduction

Based on the assumption that both obstruction and lower urinary tract symptoms (LUTS) associated with benign prostatic hyperplasia (BPH) are caused by noradrenaline stimulation of contraction-mediating, stromal α_1-adrenoceptors in the enlarged prostate, prostatic α_1-adrenoceptors have become a target for therapeutic interventions. However, considering that the size of the prostate does not correlate well with the symptoms of BPH and that LUTS typical for BPH may occur also in the absence of obstruction and in women, focus may be directed not only to the α_1-adrenoceptors in the prostate, but to α_1-adrenoceptors elsewhere in the body concerned with lower urinary tract function. In order to improve uroflow and eliminate LUTS, attempts have been made to find α_1-adrenoceptor antagonists that have effects specifically or selectively on the prostatic α_1-adrenoceptors. Such drugs have been assumed to be 'uroselective' also clinically, meaning that they should improve flow rate and eliminate LUTS without having effects on other sites in the body. However, the term uroselectivity has been used in various contexts, which may be confusing. Uroselectivity can be discussed from a receptor pharmacological, physiological, or clinical perspective, and several questions may be raised: Is uroselectivity a meaningful concept? Is it just a marketing term or has it any practical consequences?

In order to shed some light on these questions, a satellite symposium was arranged at the IVth International Consultation on BPH in Paris on July 3, 1997, entitled 'Uroselectivity: Myth or Reality?'

The first speaker, Dr. S.Z. Langer, one of the pioneers in α-adrenoceptor pharmacology, set the stage by presenting the current nomenclature of α_1-adrenoceptor subtypes, their distribution in the body, and, in particular, in the human prostate. He concluded that the α_1-adrenoceptor subtype responsible for noradrenaline-induced contraction in prostatic smooth muscle remains to be definitely established. When this receptor has been cloned and characterized, specific antagonists can be synthesized and tested, and the role of prostatic α_1-adrenoceptors for obstruction and LUTS can be clarified.

The concept of uroselectivity was discussed by Dr. K.-E. Andersson, focusing on the terms pharmacological, physiological (functional), and clinical uroselectivity. He concluded that although the terms pharmacological and functional uroselectivity may be useful in drug development, they may not be predictive of clinical effectiveness. A clinically meaningful definition can only be made in man and should consider desired drug effects on obstruction and LUTS relative to adverse effects.

Dr. D.J. Martin discussed aspects on functional uroselectivity, i.e., preferential effects on lower urinary tract smooth muscle relative to effects on blood pressure or the central nervous system. He presented data showing that pharmacological uroselectivity, i.e., selectivity for the α_{1A}-adrenoceptor in the prostate, did not predict functional uroselectivity, measured as selectivity for the bladder outlet region (intraurethral pressure) over the vasculature (blood pressure). Dr. R.S. Kirby discussed clinical uroselectivity as evidenced by results from patients treated with alfuzosin. He concluded that, because of its favourable benefit/risk ratio, alfuzosin could be classified as a clinically uroselective α_1-adrenoceptor blocker. This conclusion was supported by the data presented by Dr. B. Lukacs. His results proved the effectiveness of alfuzosin in reducing symptoms and in improving the quality of life of BPH patients during 3 years of treatment, and confirmed the favourable benefit/risk ratio of the drug.

The take-home message from the symposium was that clinical uroselectivity as defined by the International Consultation on BPH in 1995: 'desired effects on obstruction and lower urinary tract symptoms relative to adverse effects' is a meaningful one, and can be a guideline for selection of drugs for BPH that are cost-effective, safe, and that can improve the individual BPH patient's quality of life.

K.-E. Andersson, Lund
R.S. Kirby, London

KARGER
Fax +41 61 306 12 34
E-Mail karger@karger.ch
www.karger.com

This article is also accessible online at:
http://BioMedNet.com/karger

European
Urology

Eur Urol 1998;33(suppl 2):2–6

S.Z. Langer

Synthélabo Recherche (LERS), Bagneux, France

Nomenclature and State of the Art on α_1-Adrenoceptors

Key Words
α-Blockers
Benign prostatic hyperplasia
Nomenclature
Classification
Alfuzosin

Abstract

The concept of α_1-adrenoceptor subtypes was first suggested in the mid 1980s on the basis of the different affinities of certain α_1-adrenoceptor preparations for the α-adrenoceptor agonist, oxymetazoline, and the antagonists, WB4101 and phentolamine. Subsequent characterization of α_1-adrenoceptors using radioligand binding and functional studies has led to the identification of three native prazosin high-affinity α_1-adrenoceptor subtypes designated α_{1A}, α_{1B} and α_{1D}, corresponding to the three α_1-adrenoceptor subtypes (α_{1a}, α_{1b} and α_{1d}) isolated by molecular cloning techniques. Since each of these three subtypes exhibits similar affinity for the selective α_1-adrenoceptor antagonist, prazosin, [^{3}H]prazosin can be used as a convenient probe to evaluate the interaction of compounds with these adrenoceptor subtypes. Considerable clinical experience over the last few years has provided convincing evidence to support the effectiveness of α_1-adrenoceptor blockade in the treatment of bladder obstruction due to benign prostatic hyperplasia (BPH). The distribution of α_1-adrenoceptors in the human prostate tissue has shown that the predominant cloned α_1-adrenoceptor subtype characterized by RNAase protection assays corresponds to the α_{1a}-subtype, formerly classified as α_{1c}. Many of the α_1-antagonists currently prescribed in the treatment of BPH do not exhibit in vitro selectivity between α_{1a}-, α_{1b}- and α_{1d}-subtypes and yet they have good clinical tolerance in terms of low incidence of cardiovascular effects. One possibility to account for these findings is that another α_1-adrenoceptor subtype could be implicated in human prostatic smooth muscle contraction. A recent report, although confirming the presence of an α_{1a}-subtype in human prostate, suggested that an α_1-adrenoceptor subtype with lower affinity for prazosin, designated α_{1L}, which has not been cloned yet, is in fact the predominant α_1-subtype involved in the contractile response of human prostatic smooth muscle to noradrenaline.

KARGER

Fax + 41 61 306 12 34
E-Mail karger@karger.ch
www.karger.com

0302–2838/98/0338–0002$15.00/0

This article is also accessible online at:
http://BioMedNet.com/karger

Dr. S.Z. Langer
Syntélabo Recherche (LERS), BPr 110
31, avenue Paul-Vaillant-Couturier
F–92225 Bagneux (France)
Tel. +33 1 45 36 24 11, Fax +33 1 45 36 20 12

Table 1. α_1-Adrenoceptor subtypes

Native	Cloned, historical nomenclature (to be discontinued)	Cloned, new nomenclature
α_{1A}	α_{1c}	α_{1a}
α_{1B}	α_{1b}	α_{1b}
α_{1D}	α_{1a}, α_{1d}, $\alpha_{1a/d}$	α_{1d}

Introduction

The adrenoceptors belong to the superfamily of G-protein-coupled receptors and exhibit divergent affinities for many synthetic drugs. The availability of new pharmacological tools has led to a subdivision of these adrenoceptors into three separate subfamilies (α_1-, α_2-, β-adrenoceptors), each containing distinct receptor subtypes [1–3].

α_1-, α_2- and β-Adrenoceptors respond to one neurotransmitter – noradrenaline – and these receptors represent the translation effect of noradrenaline release from nerve terminals into many different tissues, e.g. the urogenital tract.

The two α-adrenoceptors can be distinguished by their relative affinities for selective agonists and antagonists [4]. Subsequently, the concept of two pharmacologically distinct subtypes of the α_1-adrenoceptors, namely α_{1A} and α_{1B}, was suggested based on their different affinities for the α-adrenoceptor agonist, oxymetazoline, and the antagonists, WB4101 and phentolamine [5].

This subtype heterogeneity was then supported by reports that the alkylating agent chlorethylclonidine [6] and the dihydropyridine calcium channel blocker, nifedipine [7] exhibited differential potencies on α_1-adrenoceptor-mediated effects.

α-Adrenoceptor Classification

Molecular cloning techniques have confirmed and extended the concept of a subfamily of α_1-adrenoceptor gene products. To date, three distinct members of the α_1-adrenoceptor subfamily (α_{1a}, α_{1b} and α_{1d}) have been cloned from different mammalian species. The α_{1b}-adrenoceptor subtype has been cloned from hamster [8], rat [9] and man [10]. Another subtype, originally given the classification α_{1c}-adrenoceptor, was identified in bovine brain [11]. In addition, a further subtype, the α_{1d}-adrenoceptor (originally given an α_{1a}-adrenoceptor nomenclature) has been cloned from rat [12, 13] and man [14].

Table 2. Cloned α_1-adrenoceptor subtypes

	Cloned α_1-adrenoceptors		
	α_{1a}	α_{1b}	α_{1d}
Transmembrane domains	7	7	7
Number of amino acid residues	466	517 (man) 515 (rat, hamster)	560
Species	man rat bovine	man rat hamster	man rat
Human chromosome location	C8	C5	C20

Unfortunately, the nomenclature used to identify the native and recombinant α_1-adrenoceptor subtypes has not been consistent, and the IUPHAR Sub-Committee on Nomenclature for Adrenoceptor has since produced a new scheme [15] (table 1).

Molecular Characterization of the Human α_1-Adrenoceptor

The three cloned α_1-adrenoceptors, α_{1a}, α_{1b} and α_{1d}, are all of the α_{1H}-type – with high affinity for prazosin – and also belong to the group of 7-transmembrane domain receptors.

A characteristic feature of these cloned α_1-adrenoceptor subfamily members is the high degree of amino acid similarity that they exhibit in their transmembrane domains (65–73% identity). In contrast, the amino acid and carboxy termini as well as the third intracellular loop sequence display marked subtype-specific differences. With respect to the human α_1-adrenoceptor, the cloned α_{1a}-subtype has 466 amino acid residues, the α_{1b}-subtype has 515 amino acid residues, and the α_{1d} has 560 amino acid residues (table 2).

Pharmacological Profiles of α_1-Adrenoceptor Subtypes

Each of the three cloned α_1-adrenoceptor subtypes (α_{1a}, α_{1b} and α_{1d}) exhibits similar affinity for the selective α_1-adrenoceptor antagonist, prazosin. As such, [^{3}H]prazosin can be used as a convenient probe to evaluate the interaction of compounds with these different subtypes. Typical

Table 3. Pharmacological profiles of [^{3}H]prazosin binding to various cloned α_1-adrenoceptor subtype membrane preparations

Compounds	pK_i – transfected α_1-adrenoceptor cell line type		
	α_{1a}	α_{1b}	α_{1d}
WB4101	10.09	8.43	9.37
Prazosin	9.73	10.18	9.71
Phentolamine	9.02	7.82	7.89
5-Methylurapidil	8.89	7.21	7.75
Oxymetazoline	7.81	6.65	6.02
Spiperone	8.65	9.04	8.30

The potencies of the drugs are expressed as the negative logarithms of their K_i values (pK_i). Data from Faure et al. [16]. α_{1a}: bovine brain; α_{1b}: hamster smooth muscle; α_{1d}: cerebral cortex.

Table 4. Affinities of cloned human α_1-adrenoceptor subtypes for α_1-adrenergic agents

Agonists	pK_i		
	α_{1a}	α_{1b}	α_{1d}
(–)Noradrenaline [21]	6.0	6.15	7.36
Methoxamine [21]	5.22	4.01	4.92
Oxymetazoline [21]	8.17	6.49	6.40

Table 5. Affinities of cloned α_1-adrenoceptor subtypes for α_1-adrenergic agents

Antagonists	pK_i		
	α_{1a}	α_{1b}	α_{1d}
Alfuzosin [16]	8.42	8.93	8.58
Prazosin [16]	9.77	9.60	10.18
5-Methylurapidil [21]	9.05	7.41	8.00
(+)Niguldipine [21]	9.13	6.66	7.40
KMD 3213 [21]	10.44	7.68	8.70
Tamsulosin [23]	10.5	9.2	10.0
BMY 7378 [24]	6.6	7.2	9.4

Table 6. Distribution of α_1-adrenoceptor (AR) subtype mRNA in human tissues

Tissue	α_1-AR mRNA molecules/ng of tissue poly(A$^+$) RNA (mean ± SEM) (n = 3)		
	α_{1a}	α_{1b}	α_{1d}
Heart	4 368 ± 720	1 044 ± 74	131 ± 17
Spleen	2 138 ± 102	5 351 ± 650	429 ± 108
Lung	955 ± 69	3 299 ± 118	792 ± 80
Prostate	1 749[a]	631 ± 287	1 724 ± 116
Urethra	90[b]	977[b]	2 267[b]

[a] n = 2.
[b] n = 1.

α_{1a}-adrenoceptor-selective agents include 5-methylurapidil, oxymetazoline, WB4101 and phentolamine and the rank order of potencies of these drugs to inhibit [^{3}H]prazosin binding to this subtype correlates as expected with their potency to inhibit [^{3}H]prazosin binding to a typical native α_{1A}-adrenoceptor tissue preparation such as rat salivary gland [16, 17]. The α_{1b}-adrenoceptor exhibits a lower affinity for 5-methylurapidil, oxymetazoline, WB4101 and phentolamine (table 3) but a higher affinity for spiperone compared to the α_{1a}- and α_{1d}-subtypes; the pharmacological profile of this α_{1b}-subtype corresponds to that of the native rat liver α_{1B}-subtype [16, 18].

Recently, selective α_{1d}-adrenoceptor compounds like BMY7378 and SKF105954 with similar affinities for the native rat aorta α_{1D}-adrenoceptor subtype have also been described [19]. Moreover, alkylation-inactivation experiments with chlorethylclonidine and SZL-49 confirm the existence of three pharmacologically distinct cloned subtypes and further illustrate the concordance between the native α_{1A}/cloned α_{1a} and native α_{1B}/cloned α_{1b} subtypes [20]. The availability of a portfolio of α_1-adrenoceptor subtype-selective antagonists will hopefully facilitate the delineation of those functional responses mediated by particular α_1-adrenoceptor subtypes.

With specific reference to the characterization of α_1-adrenoceptor subtypes seen in human tissues including the genitourinary tract, the affinity for the cloned α_1-adrenoceptors has been evaluated for different agonists, e.g. noradrenaline, methoxamine and oxymetazoline.

In general, the agonists show high affinity for the α_{1a}- and α_{1d}-subtypes. The results from pK_i values show that:

– noradrenaline shows greater affinity for the $\alpha_{1d} > \alpha_{1a} \geq \alpha_{1b}$;

– methoxamine shows lower affinity in general for the three subtypes, and

– oxymetazoline shows clear affinity for the α_{1a}-subtype compared to the α_{1b}- and α_{1d}-subtypes (table 4).

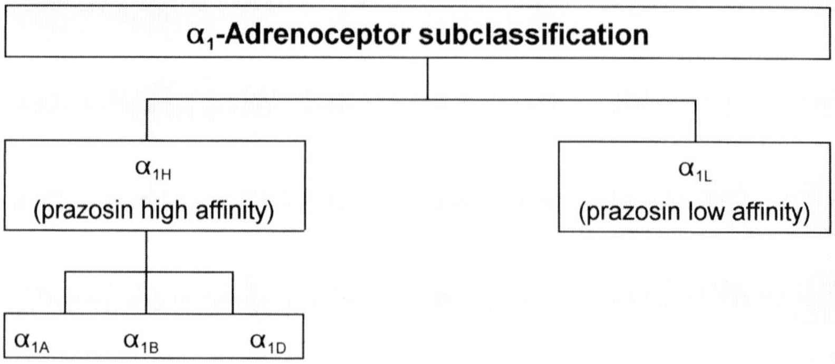

Fig. 1. α_1-Adrenoceptor subclassification.

The affinity of the cloned α_1-adrenoceptors for the different antagonists has also been evaluated (table 5). The results from pK_i values tend to show selectivity for either the α_{1a}- or α_{1d}-subtypes, e.g., 5-methylurapidil, KMD3213 and (+)niguldipine.

With specific reference to the α_1-antagonists currently employed in the treatment of benign prostatic hyperplasia (BPH), alfuzosin shows similar high affinity for the 3 subtypes α_{1a}, α_{1b} and α_{1d} and tamsulosin shows a preferential affinity for the α_{1a}- and α_{1d}-subtypes compared to the α_{1b}-subtype.

In the subclassification of α_1-adrenoceptors, one should distinguish between those which possess high affinity for prazosin (α_{1H}) and which have been cloned and expressed and whose pharmacology is well established (e.g. α_{1A}, α_{1B} and α_{1D}; fig. 1), and the α_1-subtype with low affinity for prazosin (α_{1L}), which has not been cloned yet, and may be the predominant α_1-subtype involved in the contractile response of human prostatic smooth muscle to noradrenaline [22].

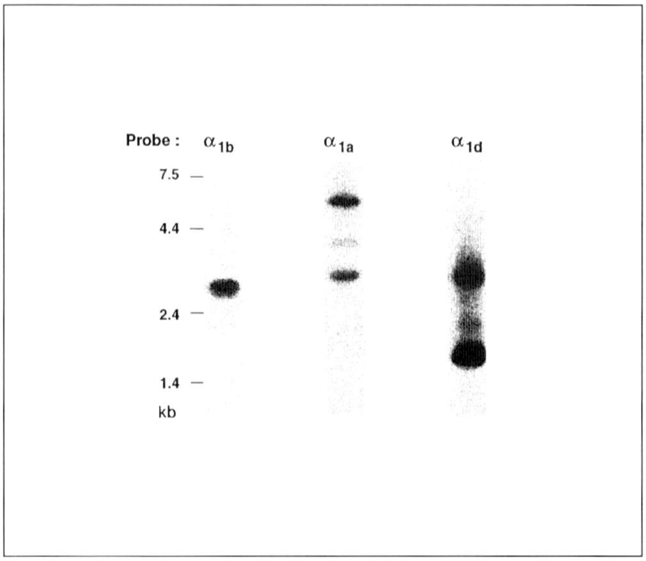

Fig. 2. Northern blot analysis of α_1-AR expression in human prostatic adenomas.

Location of α-Adrenoceptor Subtypes

Quantitative expression patterns of the messenger RNA molecules encoding the three α_1-adrenoceptor subtypes in various human tissues including the heart, spleen, lung, prostate and urethra were determined using a competitive RT-PCR approach (table 6).

These results show that the α_{1a}- and α_{1d}-subtypes are both expressed together in the prostate while in the heart the α_{1a} is predominant and in the spleen and lung, the α_{1b} is predominant. The presence of all 3 subtypes in human prostate has also been shown using Northern blot analysis (fig. 2).

In the human prostate, the predominant cloned α_1-adrenoceptor subtype characterized by RNase protection assays was shown to correspond to the α_{1a}-subtype, formerly classified as α_{1c} [25]. In addition, in situ hybridization localized this α_{1a}-mRNA for the most part to the stroma of this tissue [25]. Competitive inhibition experiments of [^{3}H]prazosin binding by selected ligands to membrane preparations of human prostate also confirmed the presence of this subtype in the tissue [26].

Discussion

Three subtypes of α_1-adrenoceptors (α_{1a}, α_{1b}, α_{1d}) have been cloned, characterized and shown to exhibit different pharmacological and tissue expression profiles. Each subtype is expressed in human prostate although in situ hybridization studies localize the α_{1a} mRNA transcripts to the stromal compartment of the prostate, and RNase protection assays suggest that this is the predominant cloned subtype. There are however conflicting studies as to whether the functional α_1-subtype in the human prostate is the α_{1A}-subtype as several antagonists selective for the α_{1A}-subtype do not block agonist responses to epinephrine and norepirephrine in the human prostate.

Recent evidence would seem to indicate the importance of the α_{1L}-subtype and that it exists in different tissues and is suspected to be present in the prostate. Once the α_{1L}-subtype has been cloned and characterized then specific antagonists can be synthesized and tested to clarify its importance in human prostate smooth muscle contraction.

References

1 Langer SZ: Presynaptic regulation of catecholamine release. Biochem Pharmacol 1974;23: 1793–1800.
2 Dubocovich ML, Langer SZ: Negative feedback regulation of noradrenaline release by nerve stimulation in the perfused cat's spleen: Differences in potency of phenoxybenzamine in blocking the pre- and post-synaptic adrenergic receptors. J Physiol 1974;237:505–519.
3 Bylund DB, Eikenberg DC, Hieble JP, Langer SZ, Lefkowitz RJ, Minneman KP, Molinoff PB, Ruffolo RR Jr, Trendelenburg U: IV International Union of Pharmacology: Nomenclature of Adrenoceptors. Pharmacol Rev 1994; 46:121–136.
4 Langer SZ: Presynaptic regulation of the release of catecholamines. Pharmacol Rev 1981; 32:337–362.
5 Morrow AL, Creese I : Characterization of α_1-adrenergic receptor subtypes in rat brain: A reevaluation of ^{3}H-WB4101 and ^{3}H-prazosin binding. Mol Pharmacol 1986;29:321–330.
6 Minneman KP, Han C, Abel PW: Comparison of α_1-adrenergic receptor subtypes distinguished by chlorethylclonidine and WB4101. Mol Pharmacol 1988;33:509–514.
7 Han C, Abel PW, Minneman KP: α_1-Adrenoceptor subtypes linked to different mechanisms for increasing intracellular Ca^{2+} in smooth muscle. Nature 1987;329–333.
8 Cotecchia S, Schwinn DA, Randall RR, Lefkowitz RJ, Caron MG, Kobilka BK: Molecular cloning and expression of the cDNA for the hamster α_1-adrenoceptor. Proc Natl Acad Sci USA 1988;85:7159–7163.
9 Voigt MM, Kispert J, Chin H: Sequence of a rat brain cDNA encoding an alpha-1B adrenergic receptor. Nucleic Acids Res 1990;18:1053.
10 Ramarao CS, Denker JMK, Perez DM, Gaivin RJ, Riek RP, Graham RM, Genomic organization and expression of the human α_{1b}-adrenergic receptor. J Biol Chem 1992;267:21936–21945.
11 Schwinn DA, Lomasney JW, Lorenz W, Szklut PJ, Fremeau RT, Yang-Feng TL, Caron MG, Lefkowitz RJ, Cotecchia S: Molecular cloning and expression of the cDNA for a novel α_1-adrenergic receptor subtype. J Biol Chem 1990; 265:8183–8189.
12 Lomasney JW, Cotechia S, Lorenz W, Leung WY, Schwinn DA, Yang-Feng TL, Brownstein M, Lefkowitz RJ, Caron M: Molecular cloning and expression of the cDNA for the α_{1A}-adrenergic receptor. J Biol Chem 1991;266:6365–6369.
13 Perez DM, Piascik MT, Graham RM, Solution-phase library screening for the identification of rare clones: Isolation of an α_{1d}-adrenergic receptor cDNA. Mol Pharmacol 1991;40: 876–883.
14 Bruno JFJ, Whittaker J, Song J, Berelowitz M: Molecular cloning and sequencing of a cDNA encoding a human α_{1A}-adrenergic receptor. Biochem Biophys Res Commun 1991;179: 1485–1490.
15 Hieble JP, Bylund DB, Clarke DI, Eikenberg DC, Langer SZ, Lefkowitz RJ, Minneman KP, Ruffolo RR Jr: Recommendations of nomenclature of α_1-adrenoceptors: Consensus update. Pharmacol Rev 1995;47:267–270.
16 Faure C, Pimoule C, Arbilla S, Langer SZ, Graham D : Expression of α_1-adrenoceptor subtypes in rat tissues: Implications for α_1-adrenoceptor classification. Eur J Pharmacol Mol Pharmacol Sect 1994;268:141–149.
17 Michel AD, Loury DN, Whiting RL : Identification of single α_1-adrenoceptor corresponding to the α_{1A}-subtype in rat submaxillary gland. Br J Pharmacol 1989;98:883–889.
18 Han C, Abel PW, Minneman KP: Heterogeneity of α_1-adrenergic receptors revealed by chlorethylclonidine. Mol Pharmacol 1987;32:505–510.
19 Goetz AS, King HK, Ward SDC, True TA, Rimele TJ, Saussy DL: BMY7378 is a selective antagonist of the D subtype of α_1-adrenoceptors. Eur J Pharmacol 1995;272:R5–R6.
20 Pimoule C, Langer SZ, Graham D : Further evidence that the classical α_{1A}- and the cloned α_{1c}-adrenoceptors are the same subtype. Eur J Pharmacol Mol Pharmacol Sect 1995;290:49–53.
21 Shibata K, Foglar R, Horie K, Obika K, Stamoto A, Ogawa S, Tsujimoto G: KMD-3213, a novel potent, α_{1a}-adrenoceptor selective antagonist: Characterization using recombinant human α_1-adrenoceptors and native tissues Mol Pharmacol 1995;48:250–258.
22 Muramatsu I, Oshita M, Ohmura T, Kigoshi S, Akino H, Gobora M, Okada K: Pharmacological characterization of α_1-adrenoceptor subtypes in the human prostate: Functional and binding studies. Br J Urol 1994;74:572–578.
23 Foglar R, Shibata K, Horier K, Hirasawa A, Tsujimoto G: Use of recombinant α_1-adrenoceptors to characterize subtype selectivity of drugs for the treatment of prostatic hypertrophy. Eur J Pharmacol Mol Pharmacol Sect 1995;288:201–207.
24 Wetzel JM, Micro SW, Forray C, Borden LA, Branchek TA, Gluchowski C: Discovery of α_{1a}-adrenergic receptor antagonists based on the L-type G2T channel antagonist niguldipine. J Med Chem 1995;38:1579–1581.
25 Price DT, Schwinn DA, Lomasney JW, Allen LF, Caron MG, Lefkowitz RJ: Identification, quantification, and localization of mRNA for three distinct alpha1 adrenergic receptor subtypes in human prostate. J Urol 1993;150:546–551.
26 Faure C, Pimoule C, Vallancien G, Langer SZ, Graham D : Identification of α_1-adrenoceptor subtypes present in the human prostate. Life Sci 1994;54:1595–1605.

European Urology

Eur Urol 1998;33(suppl 2):7–11

Karl-Erik Andersson

Department of Clinical Pharmacology, Lund University Hospital, Lund, Sweden

The Concept of Uroselectivity

Key Words
Benign prostatic hyperplasia
Bladder outflow obstruction
Blood pressure
α_1-Adrenoceptor antagonists
Lower urinary tract

Abstract

α_1-Adrenoceptor antagonists have been shown to decrease both the voiding and storage symptoms of benign prostatic hyperplasia (BPH). Based on the assumption that these symptoms can be attributed to the consequences of the increase in outflow resistance caused by noradrenaline stimulation of stromal α_1-adrenoceptors in the enlarged prostate, prostatic α_1-adrenoceptors have become a target for therapeutic interventions. In some patients, α_1-adrenoceptor antagonists in common clinical use produce intolerable side effects which may be attributed to action on non-prostatic α_1-adrenoceptors. Therefore, attempts have been made to find α_1-adrenoceptor antagonists that have selective effects on the prostate ('uroselective' agents), to maintain efficacy in uroflow and eliminate adverse effects. The term uroselectivity has been used in various contexts, but drugs may be discussed as uroselective from a receptor pharmacological, physiological, or clinical perspective. Provided that the α_1-adrenoceptor subtype in the prostate, bladder neck and urethra is uniform, unique, and cannot be found in other parts of the body, drugs with selectivity for this receptor could be called uroselective. However, available evidence suggests that (1) more than one α_1-adrenoceptor subtype can be found in the lower urinary tract, and that the main α_1-adrenoceptor mediating contraction still remains to be definitely defined; (2) the receptor(s) is (are) most probably not unique to the lower urinary tract, and (3) α_1-adrenoceptor sites outside the prostate (with still undefined subtypes) may contribute to the lower urinary tract symptoms of BPH. Therefore, it does not seem possible to define uroselectivity in terms of selectivity for the α_1-adrenoceptor(s) occurring in the prostate. Several animal models have been developed where the potency order of effects of various α_1-adrenoceptor antagonists on blood pressure and urethral pressure have been measured simultaneously. Such models can be useful when screening drugs that may be developed for therapeutic use, but they also have limitations, since side effects that may be dose limiting clinically are not always related to a decrease in blood pressure. Certainly, a drug may be said to have physiological or functional uroselectivity if it lowers outflow resistance more effectively than it affects other defined physiological functions. A clinically meaningful definition of uroselectivity can only be made in man and considers desired effects on obstruction and lower urinary tract symptoms relative to adverse effects.

Background

Obstructive and irritative symptoms (table 1) associated with benign prostatic hyperplasia (BPH) have traditionally been linked to the prostate. Obstructive symptoms have been attributed to two factors [Caine, 1986]: the physical mass of the enlarged gland (the static component), and the tone of the smooth muscle of the prostatic stroma (the dynamic component). Irritative symptoms, on the other hand, have been more closely associated with the bladder dysfunction produced by the increased outflow resistance. The connections between BPH, bladder outflow obstruction and symptoms are unclear, however [Shapiro and Lepor, 1995]. Both obstructive and irritative symptoms have been shown to be common also in women [Jollys et al., 1993; Lepor and Machi, 1993], and many

KARGER
Fax + 41 61 306 12 34
E-Mail karger@karger.ch
www.karger.com

0302–2838/98/0338–0007$15.00/0

This article is also accessible online at:
http://BioMedNet.com/karger

Dr. Karl-Erik Andersson
Department of Urology, University of Virginia Health Sciences Center
PO Box 422
Charlottesville, VA 22908 (USA)
Tel. +1 (804) 924 2224, Fax +1 (804) 982 36 52
E-Mail ka3x@virginia.edu

Table 1. Lower urinary tract symptoms associated with BPH

Voiding symptoms	Filling symptoms
Hesitancy	Urgency
Intermittency	Urinary frequency
Decreased force of the urinary stream	Sense of incomplete voiding
Dribbling retention	Nocturia
	Incontinence

Table 2. α_1-Adrenoceptor antagonists and lower urinary tract symptoms in BPH – possible sites of action

Prostate
Urethra and trigone
Detrusor
Spinal cord
Supraspinal structures
Peripheral ganglia

patients who have undergone prostatectomy, which should relieve obstruction, still experience persistent irritative symptoms. Abrams [1994] therefore suggested that 'lower urinary tract symptoms' (LUTS), which neutrally describes the symptoms of the patients, should be used instead of 'prostatism', and introduced the terms 'voiding' and 'filling' to replace 'obstructive' and 'irritative' symptoms, respectively.

It is logical to assume that prostatic α-adrenoceptors should be responsible for at least part of the LUTS associated with BPH. However, the well-documented beneficial effects of α_1-adrenoceptor antagonists on the symptoms of BPH [Eri and Tveter, 1995; Chapple, 1996; Jardin et al., 1996; Andersson et al., 1997], even in the absence of outflow obstruction, give support to the involvement of extraprostatic α_1-adrenoceptors in the pathogenesis of LUTS (table 2). Indeed, there is evidence for the involvement of α-adrenoceptors in the spinal control of both the sympathetic and somatic (filling), as well as the parasympathetic (voiding) efferent activity to the lower urinary tract [Andersson et al., 1997].

In approximately 10% of patients, the use of α_1-adrenoceptor antagonists in common clinical use (alfuzosin, doxazosin, tamsulosin, terazosin) has been limited by intolerable side effects – i.e., dizziness, headache, asthenia, nasal congestion, and orthostatic hypotension – which may be attributed to an action on non-prostatic α_1-adrenoceptors. To avoid these side effects, attempts have been made to find α_1-adrenoceptor antagonists that have selective effects on the prostatic α_1-adrenoceptors, assuming that they should be 'uroselective' also in terms of relieving LUTS without systemic side effects. The criteria for 'uroselectivity', however, have not been previously established, and the term has been used in various contexts, which may be confusing. Drugs may be 'uroselective' from a receptor pharmacological, physiological, or clinical perspective.

Pharmacological Uroselectivity

α_1-Adrenoceptors

Multiple α_1-adrenoceptor subtypes have been identified, which could offer the opportunity to target the prostate selectively. Receptor cloning and pharmacological studies in human tissues have revealed the existence of at least three subtypes of the α_1-adrenoceptor [Bylund et al., 1994; Hieble et al., 1995; Michel et al., 1995; Graham et al., 1996], and consensus has been reached on classification and nomenclature [Hieble et al., 1995]. Current α_1-adrenoceptor classification recognises three native subtypes that have been designated as α_{1A}, α_{1B} and α_{1D}. The cloned counterparts are now termed α_{1a}, α_{1b}, and α_{1d}. These three subtypes are classified as α_{1H}-adrenoceptors for having high affinity for prazosin. It is important to be aware of the impact of this re-classification when reviewing historical data, as many different classifications have been used in the derivation of the conclusions. There is increasing evidence that an additional α_1-adrenoceptor subtype with low affinity for prazosin (α_{1L}), which is not yet fully characterized, may occur in, for example, vascular and prostatic smooth muscle (see below).

α_1-Adrenoceptors in the Prostate and Urethra

Nerves containing adrenergic, cholinergic and non-adrenergic, non-cholinergic transmitters or mediator-producing enzymes supply the smooth muscles of the prostate capsule and the trabecular tissue around the ducts [Dail, 1993; Hedlund et al., 1997]. However, the adrenergic nerves are considered responsible for prostatic smooth muscle tone by releasing noradrenaline, which stimulates contraction-mediating α-adrenoceptors [Caine et al., 1975]. Approximately 50% of the total urethral pressure in BPH patients may be due to α-adrenoceptor-mediated muscle tone [Appell et al., 1980; Furuya et al., 1982]. Although both α_1- and α_2-adrenoceptors can be identified within the human prostate, the contractile effects of noradrenaline are mediated primarily by α_1-adrenoceptors [see Andersson et al., 1997].

In BPH, there may be an increased density of prostatic α_1-adrenoceptors [Yamada et al., 1987; Nasu et al., 1996) localised to the stroma [Chapple et al., 1989; Kobayashi et al., 1993; Nasu et al., 1996]. The distinct α_1-adrenoceptor subtypes (α_{1H} and α_{1L}) have been suggested to be present in the human prostate [Muramatsu et al., 1994; Maruyama et al. 1996]. Although all the three high-affinity α_1-adrenoceptor subtypes found in molecular cloning studies have been identified in prostatic stromal tissue [Andersson et al., 1997], the α_{1a}-subtype was found to predominate, representing about 60–85% of the α_1-adrenoceptor population.

The α_{1A}-adrenoceptor was reported to mediate the contractile response of the human prostate in vitro [Forray et al., 1994; Marshall et al., 1995]. However, an important contribution of other subtypes cannot be excluded. Thus, Ford et al. [1995, 1996a] found that the α_{1A}-adrenoceptor may not mediate contractile responses to noradrenaline, and suggested the α_{1L}-adrenoceptor as a candidate. Findings by Kenny et al. [1996] support the view that the α_{1L}-adrenoceptor, which appears to share many of the characteristics of an α_{1A}-adrenoceptor, mediates the contractile response of the human prostate. On the other hand, it has also been suggested that the α_{1A}- and α_{1L}-adrenoceptor may represent distinct pharmacological sites of the same receptor [Ford et al., 1996b].

α_1-Adrenoceptors in the Detrusor

In the detrusor muscle of most species, including humans, relaxation-mediating β-adrenoceptors normally dominate over contraction-mediating α-adrenoceptors, and the effect of drugs stimulating α-adrenoceptors is small. Thus, the normal response to noradrenaline is relaxation. However, this may change with outflow obstruction. Perlberg and Caine [1982] assessed whether the response to noradrenaline changed in the hypertrophic bladder, and found that in strips taken from hypertrophic bladders, noradrenaline-induced β-adrenoceptor-mediated relaxation became an α-adrenoceptor-mediated contraction in almost one fourth of the patients. This change in the response of the bladder to noradrenaline was also reflected in the symptoms. Patients who had a contractile reaction to noradrenaline had symptoms of bladder overactivity. Apparently, such a change in the noradrenaline response may play a role in the production of symptoms. However, Smith and Chapple [1994] studied α_1-adrenoceptor functions in strips from obstructed bladders. Only 5 of 72 strips responded to phenylephrine. These results are not in agreement with the view that α-adrenoceptor stimulation during storage contributes to contraction. Thus, changes occur in the balance between β- and α-adrenoceptor functions, but it is not known what this really means as concerns bladder symptoms, particularly storage symptoms.

Walden et al. [1997] reported a predominance of α_{1a}-adrenoceptor protein in the human bladder dome, trigone and bladder base, and suggested that the α_{1A}-adrenoceptor subtype predominates functionally in this region. However, the number of α_1-adrenoceptors in the human detrusor is extremely small [Goepel et al., 1997], and their importance for bladder contraction under normal conditions may be questioned.

α_1-Adrenoceptors in Central and Peripheral Nervous Structures

Noradrenaline-containing projections supplying sympathetic and parasympathetic nuclei in the lumbosacral spinal cord have been demonstrated [de Groat et al., 1993], and bladder activation through bulbospinal pathways may involve excitatory α_1-adrenoceptors. Central, facilitatory α_1-adrenoceptors, tonically active in both the sympathetic and somatic neural control of the lower urinary tract, have been demonstrated in the cat [Danuser and Thor, 1995; Ramage and Wyllie, 1995]. In both normal rats and rats with bladder hypertrophy secondary to outflow obstruction, Ishizuka et al. [1996] reported that doxazosin may act at the level of the spinal cord and ganglia, thereby reducing the activity in the parasympathetic nerves to the bladder, an effect which was more pronounced in rats with bladder hypertrophy than in normal rats. If such actions are relevant to the effects of α_1-adrenoceptor antagonists in humans, extraprostatic α_1-adrenoceptors may be relevant targets for drugs meant for the treatment of LUTS.

In animal models, facilitatory α_1-adrenoceptors have been demonstrated on cholinergic neurons in the vesical ganglia of the cat [Keast et al., 1990], and on cholinergic terminals in the rat bladder [Somogyi et al., 1995]. An effect of α_1-adrenoceptor antagonists at the ganglionic and/or prejunctional level, leading to a decrease of acetylcholine release cannot be excluded.

α_1-Adrenoceptors in the Cardiovascular System

Of particular interest is the involvement of α_1-adrenoceptor subtypes in vascular control. Although species- and vessel-dependent, α_{1A}-, α_{1B}-, α_{1D}-, and α_{1L}-adrenoceptors all seem to subserve the contractile response in vascular tissue [Hatano et al., 1994, Kohno et al., 1994; Kenny et al., 1995; Muramatsu et al., 1995; Vargas and Gorman, 1995]. On this basis, one could assume that cardiovascular homeostasis depends on all of the multiple subtypes, albeit to varying extents.

Physiological Uroselectivity

Drugs which decrease outflow resistance without affecting blood pressure would obviously be of therapeutic interest. The potency order of effects of various α_1-adrenoceptor antagonists on the pressures in the urethra has been defined in several animal models. This has then been related to blood pressure changes in the same animal [Martin et al., 1996, 1997; Andersson et al., 1997]. Although such models may have some predictive value, they also have limitations. Thus, results obtained in one animal species may differ from those obtained in another, and it has not been established which animal model is the most relevant to effects in humans. Since side effects that may be dose limiting clinically are not always cardiovascular, but may originate from the central nervous system, e.g, drowsiness and dizziness, and since such effects cannot always be studied in animals, animal models may not adequately predict clinical usefulness.

Clinical Uroselectivity

A clinically relevant definition of uroselectivity can only be made in man. It is known that effects of α_1-adrenoceptor antagonists on blood pressure are more pronounced in hypertensive subjects than in normotensive ones. Theoretically, a drug could affect blood pressure in a hypertensive subject before it has any noticable effects on the urethra, i.e., the drug has no 'uroselectivity'. The same drug may reduce outflow resistance in a normotensive subject without any effects on blood pressure, i.e., the drug is 'uroselective'. Also, pharmacokinetic properties may contribute to apparent differences between drugs in effects on different organ systems. It is therefore necessary to have a broad definition of clinical uroselectivity, taking into account that the clinical endpoints, i.e. outflow obstruction, as defined urodynamically, LUTS, and adverse effects may be more or less independent. Thus, a clinical therapeutic index may be defined, describing in relative terms the ratio between the dose required for desired therapeutic action and the dose producing side effects. Such a definition of uroselectivity is the one suggested by the 3rd International Consultation on Benign Prostatic Hyperplasia in 1995: 'desired effects on obstruction and lower urinary tract symptoms related to adverse effects'. It should be noted that clinical uroselectivity defined in this way is not an all or none phenomenon.

Conclusions

A drug may be uroselective in the sense that it has a preference for the α_1-adrenoceptors in the prostate, or that, in an animal model, it can affect the prostate and urethra without affecting, e.g., blood pressure. Since there are α_1-adrenoceptors in the urethra, trigone, detrusor, spinal cord, supraspinal structures and peripheral ganglia, whose contribution to the symptoms of BPH remains unknown, and whose subtypes have not been determined, such definition of uroselectivity may not be very meaningful from a clinical point of view. A clinically meaningful definition of uroselectivity can only be made in man and considers desired effects on obstruction and lower urinary tract symptoms relative to adverse effects.

References

Abrams P: New words for old: Urinary tract symptoms for 'prostatism'. Br Med J 1994;308:929–930.

Andersson KE, Lepor H, Wyllie M: Prostatic α_1-adrenoceptors and uroselectivity. Prostate 1997;30:202–215.

Appell RA, England HR, Hussell AR, McGuire EJ: The effect of epidural anesthesia on the urethral closure pressure profile in patients with prostatic enlargement. J Urol 1980;124:410–411.

Bylund DB, Eikenberg DC, Hieble JP, Langer SZ, Lefkowitz RJ, Minneman KP, Molinoff PB, Ruffolo R Jr, Trendelenburg U: International Union of Pharmacology Nomenclature of Adrenoceptors. Pharmacol Rev 1994;46:121–136.

Caine M: The present role of alpha-adrenergic blockers in the treatment of benign prostatic hypertrophy. J Urol 1986;136:1–4.

Caine M, Raz S, Zeigler M: Adrenergic and cholinergic receptors in the human prostate, prostatic capsule and bladder neck. Br J Urol 1975;47: 193–202.

Chapple CR: Selective α_1-adrenoceptor antagonists in benign prostatic hyperplasia: Rationale and clinical experience. Eur Urol 1996;29:129–144.

Chapple CR, Aubrey ML, James S, Greengrass P M, Burnstock G, Turner-Warwick RT, Milroy EJ, Davey MJ: Characterisation of human prostatic adrenoceptors using pharmacology receptor binding and localisation. Br J Urol 1989;63:487–496.

Dail WG: Autonomic innervation of male reproductive genitalia; in Maggi CA (ed): The Autonomic Nervous System. London, Harwood Academic Publishers, 1993, vol 6, chapter 9: Nervous Control of the Urogenital System, pp 69–101.
Danuser H, Thor K: Inhibition of central sympathetic and somatic outflow to the lower urinary tract of the cat by the α_1-adrenergic receptor antagonist prazosin. J Urol 1995;153:1308–1312.
Eri LM, Tveter KJ: α-Blockade in the treatment of symptomatic benign prostatic hyperplasia. J Urol 1995;154:923–934.
Ford APDW, Arredondo NF, Blue DR Jr, Bonhaus DW, Kava MS, Williams TJ, Vimont RL, Zhu QM, Pfister JR, Clarke DE: Do alpha-1A (alpha-1C)-adrenoceptors (AR) mediate prostatic smooth muscle contraction in man? Studies with a novel, selective alpha-1A-AR antagonist, RS 17053. Br J Pharmacol 1995;114:24P.
Ford APDW, Arredondo NF, Blue DR, Bonhaus DW, Jasper J, Kava MS, Lesnick J, Pfister JR, Shieh IA, Williams TJ, McNeal JE, Stamey TA, Clarke DE: (N-[2-(2-Cyclopropylmethoxyphenoxy)ethyl-5-chloro-α, α-dimethyl-1H-indole-3-ethanamine hydrochloride), a selective α_{1A}-adrenoceptor antagonist, displays low affinity for functional α_1-adrenoceptors in human prostate: Implications for adrenoceptor classification. Mol Pharmacol 1996a;49:209–215.
Ford APDW, Daniels DV, Chang DJ, Diaz MR, Gever JR, Jasper J, Lesnick J, Clarke DE: The putative α_{1L} receptor (AR): A distinct pharmacological state of the α_{1A}-adrenoceptor? Br J Pharmacol 1996b;118:29P.
Forray C, Bard JA, Wetzel JM, Chiu G, Shapiro E, Tang R, Lepor H, Hartig PR, Weinshank RL, Branchek TA, Gluchowski C: The α_1-adrenergic receptor that mediates smooth muscle contraction in human prostate has the pharmacological properties of the cloned human α_1c subtype. Mol Pharmacol 1994;45:703–708.
Furuya S, Kumamoto Y, Yokoyama E, Tsukamoto T, Izumi T, Abiko Y: Alpha-adrenergic activity and urethral pressure in prostatic zone in benign prostatic hypertrophy. J Urol 1982;128:836–839.
Goepel M, Wittmann A, Rubben H, Michel MC: Comparison of adrenoceptor subtype expression in porcine and human bladder and prostate. Urol Res 1997;25:199–206.
Graham RM, Perez DM, Hwa J, Piascik MT: α_1-Adrenergic receptor subtypes. Molecular structure, function, and signaling. Circ Res 1996;78:737–749.
de Groat WC, Booth AM, Yoshimura N: Neurophysiology of micturition and its modification in animal models of human disease; in Maggi CA (ed): The Autonomic Nervous System. London, Harwood Academic Publishers, 1993, vol 6, chap 8: Nervous Control of the Urogenital System, pp 227–289.
Hatano A, Takahashi H, Tamaki M, Komeyama T, Koizumi T, Takeda M: Pharmacological evidence of distinct α_1-adrenoceptor subtypes mediating the contraction of human prostatic urethra and peripheral artery. Br J Urol 1994;113:723–728.
Hedlund P, Ekström P, Larsson B, Alm P, Andersson K-E: Heme oxygenase and NO$^-$ synthase in the human prostate – relation to adrenergic, cholinergic and peptide-containing nerves. J Auton Nerv Syst 1997;63:115–126.
Hieble JP, Bylund DB, Clarke DE, Eikenberg DC, Langer SZ, Lefkowitz RJ, Minneman KP, Ruffolo RR Jr: International Union of Pharmacology X. Recommendation for nomenclature of α_1-adrenoceptors: Consensus update. Pharmacol Rev 1995;47:267–270.
Ishizuka O, Persson K, Mattiasson A, Naylor A, Wyllie M, Andersson K-E: Micturition in conscious rats with and without outlet obstruction: Role of spinal $\alpha_1$adrenoceptors. Br J Pharmacol 1996;117:962–966.
Jardin A, Andersson K-E, Caine M, Chapple C, El-Hilali K, Hertle L, Kawabe R, Kirby R, Lepor H, Pool J: α-Blockers therapy in benign prostatic hyperplasia; in Cockett ATK, Khoury S, Aso Y, Chatelain C, Denis L, Griffiths K, Murphy GSCI (eds): The Third International Consultation on Benign Prostatic Hyperplasia (BPH). 1996, pp 527–564.
Jollys JV, Jollys JC, Wilson J, Donovan J, Nanchamel K, Abrams P: Does sexual equality extend to urinary symptoms? Neurourol Urodyn, 1993;12:391–392.
Keast JR, Kawatani,M, de Groat WC: Sympathetic modulation of cholinergic transmission in cat vesical ganglia is mediated by α_1- and α2-adrenoceptors. Am J Physiol 1990;258:R44-R50.
Kenny BA, Chalmers DH, Philpott PC, Naylor AM: Characterisation of an α_{1D} adrenoceptors mediating the contractile response of rat aorta to noradrenaline. Br J Pharmacol, 1995;115:981–986.
Kenny BA, Miller AM, Williamson IJR, O'Connell J, Chalmers DH, Naylor AM: Evaluation of the pharmacological selectivity profile of α_1 adrenoceptor antagonists at prostatic α_1 adrenoceptors: Binding, functional and in vivo studies. Br J Pharmacol 1996;118:871–878.
Kobayashi S, Tang R, Shapiro E, Lepor H: Characterization and localization of prostatic alphaα_1 adrenoceptors using radioligand binding on slide-mounted tissue section. J Urol 1993;150:2002–2006.
Kohno Y, Saito H, Takita M, Kigoshi S, Muramatsu I: Heterogeneity of α_1-adrenoceptor subtypes involved in adrenergic contractions of dog blood vessels. Br J Pharmacol 1994;112:1167–1173.
Lepor H, Machi G: Comparison of the AUA symptom index in unselected males and females between 55 and 79 years of age. Urology 1993;42:36–40.
Marshall I, Burt RP, Chapple CR: Noradrenaline contractions of human prostate mediated by α_{1A}-(α_{1c}-)adrenoceptor subtype. Br J Pharmacol 1995;115:781–786.
Martin D, Lluel P, Jammes D, Philippo P, Angel I: α_1-Adrenoceptor selectivity is not predictive of uroselectivity – evaluation by simultaneous assessment of the urethral and blood pressures in conscious male rats (abstract 53). Eur J Urol 1996;30(suppl 2).
Martin DJ, Lluel P, Guillot E, Coste A, Jammes D, Philippo P, Angel I: Comparative alpha-1 adrenoceptor subtype selectivity and functional uroselectivity of alpha-1 adrenoceptor antagonists. J Pharmacol Exp Ther 1997;282:228–235.
Maruyama K, Fukutomi J, Chiba T, Yamaguchi M, Takeda M, Hattori K, Nagatomo T: Two distinct α_1-adrenoceptor subtypes in the human prostate: Assessment by radioligand binding assay using ^{3}H-prazosin. Gen Pharmacol 1996;27:1377–1381.
Michel MC, Kenny B, Schwinn DA: Classification of α_1 adrenoceptors. Naunyn Schmiedeberg's Arch Pharmacol 1995;352:1–10.
Muramatsu I, Ohmura T, Hashimoto S, Oshita M: Functional subclassification of vascular α_1-adrenoceptors. Pharmacol Commun 1995;6:23–28.
Muramatsu I, Oshita M, Ohmura T, Kigoshi S, Akino H, Okada K: Pharmacological characterisation of α_1 adrenoceptor subtypes in the human prostate; functional and binding studies. Br J Urol 1994;74:572–578.
Nasu K, Moriyama N, Kawabe K, Tsujimoto G, Murai M, Tanaka T, et al: Quantification and distribution of α_1-adrenoceptor subtype mRNAs in human prostate: Comparison of benign hypertrophied tissue and non-hypertrophied tissue. Br J Pharmacol 1996;119:797–803.
Perlberg S, Caine M: Adrenergic response of bladder muscle in prostatic obstruction. Urology 1982;20:524–537.
Ramage AG, Wyllie MG: A comparison of the effects of doxazosin and terazosin on the spontaneous sympathetic drive to the bladder and related organs in anesthetized cats. Eur J Pharmacol 1995;294:645–650.
Shapiro E, Lepor H: Pathophysiology of clinical benign prostatic hyperplasia. Urol Clin N Am 1995;22:285–290.
Smith DJ, Chapple CR: In vitro response of human bladder smooth muscle in unstable obstructed male bladders: A study of pathophysiological causes. Neurourol Urodyn 1994;13:414–415.
Somogyi GT, Tanowitz M, de Groat WC: Prejunctional facilitatory α_1-adrenoceptorsin the rat urinary bladder. Br J Pharmacol 1995;114:1710–1716.
Vargas HM, Gorman AJ: Vascular alpha-1 adrenergic receptor subtypes in the regulation of arterial pressure. Life Sci 1995;57:2291–2308.
Walden P, Durkin M, Lepor H, Wetzel JM, Gluchowski C, Gustafson E: Localization of mRNA and receptor binding sites for the α_{1a}-adrenoceptor in the rat, monkey and human urinary bladder and prostate. J Urol 1997;57:1032–1038.
Yamada S, Ashizawa N, Ushijima H, Nakayama K, Hayashi E, Honda K: Alpha-1 adrenoceptors in human prostate: Characterization and alteration in benign prostatic hypertrophy. J Pharmacol Exp Ther 1987;242:326–330.

European Urology

Eur Urol 1998;33(suppl 2):12–18

Functional Uroselectivity

D.J. Martin
I. Angel
S. Arbilla

Internal Medicine Research,
Synthélabo Recherche, Rueil-Malmaison,
France

Key Words
α_1-Adrenoceptor blockers
Functional uroselectivity
Benign prostatic hyperplasia

Abstract
α_1-Adrenoceptors mediating sympathetic tone to smooth muscle cells are located within the prostatic tissue, bladder base and in the proximal urethra, but are also widely distributed within a large number of tissues, especially the vascular beds and the central nervous system. Compounds clinically used in the symptomatic treatment of benign prostatic hyperplasia must therefore exhibit functional uroselectivity. This means that they should preferentially act on the lower urinary tract rather than the vasculature or central nervous system. Few clinically used α_1-adrenoceptor antagonists show selectivity for the $\alpha_{1a/A}$-adrenoceptor subtype, whereas most of them have similar affinities for the three cloned subtypes (α_{1a}-, α_{1b}- and α_{1d}-adrenoceptors). Recent data from in vitro studies assessing pharmacological uroselectivity and from in vivo models evaluating functional uroselectivity challenged the relevance of the affinity or the selectivity for a known α_1-adrenoceptor subtype in predicting functional uroselectivity. They suggest instead that another subtype, like the α_{1L}-adrenoceptor, might be functionally involved. In conclusion, the actual state of knowledge on α_1-adrenoceptor subtype distribution and function, does not support a role of pharmacological uroselectivity in predicting functional uroselectivity. Furthermore, functional uroselectivity can be achieved in the absence of selectivity for the α_1-adrenoceptor subtypes described so far.

Introduction

α_1-Adrenoceptors are present in the proximal urethra, trigone and bladder neck but are scarcer in the vesical tissue [1, 2]. Blockade of these receptors by α_1-adrenoceptor antagonists will therefore reduce sympathetic tone at different levels of the lower urinary tract and consequently decrease bladder outlet obstruction [3, 4]. As α_1-adrenoceptors are widely distributed in a large number of tissues, including the vascular beds and the central nervous system, compounds clinically used in the symptomatic treatment of benign prostatic hyperplasia (BPH) must therefore exhibit uroselectivity. This means that they are expected to act preferentially at the level of the lower urinary tract tissues rather than the vasculature or the central nervous system. At present, uroselectivity is defined ac-

KARGER
Fax + 41 61 306 12 34
E-Mail karger@karger.ch
www.karger.com

0302–2838/98/0338–0012$15.00/0

This article is also accessible online at:
http://BioMedNet.com/karger

D.J. Martin
Urology Group, Internal Medicine Research, Synthélabo Recherche
10, rue des Carrières
F–92504 Rueil-Malmaison (France)
Tel. +33 1 41 39 13 71, Fax +33 1 41 39 13 05

Table 1. Affinities of various α_1-adrenoceptor antagonists for the cloned α_1-adrenoceptors and their calculated selectivity ratios (expressed as negative log of the pK_i difference)

Compounds	Affinities for human cloned adrenoceptors (pK_i)			Selectivity ratios	
	α_{1a}	α_{1b}	α_{1d}	α_{1a}/α_{1b}	α_{1a}/α_{1d}
5-Me-urapidil [17]	8.68	6.76	7.91	83.2	0.1
RS-17053 [13]	8.90	7.10	7.20	63	50
SB 216469 [33]	9.75	8.41	9.17	21.9	0.2
WB4101 [17]	9.41	8.34	9.04	11.8	0.2
Tamsulosin [18]	9.70	8.90	9.80	6.3	0.2
Prazosin [17]	9.70	9.60	9.50	1.23	1.3
Alfuzosin [17]	8.20	8.53	8.40	0.5	1.4
Doxazosin [17]	8.56	8.98	8.78	0.4	1.6
Terazosin [17]	8.16	8.71	8.46	0.3	1.8

cording to pharmacological, functional (physiological) and clinical criteria [5].

- Pharmacological uroselectivity refers to preferential affinity of drugs for a receptor specifically distributed in the lower urinary tract.
- Functional (physiological) uroselectivity is characterized by a preferential effect on urethral pressure without significant effects either on the cardiovascular or central nervous systems.
- Clinical uroselectivity corresponds to desired effects on obstruction and lower urinary tract symptoms relative to adverse effects.

This paper presents recent experimental data on the pharmacological profile and functional uroselectivity of available α_1-adrenoceptor antagonists.

Is Affinity or Selectivity for an α_1-Adrenoceptor Subtype Predictive of in vitro Tissue Relaxant Efficacy?

Since the identification and characterization of the α-adrenoceptor subtypes [6], the classification of α_1-adrenoceptors has considerably evolved. Currently, three α_1-adrenoceptor subtypes, designated α_{1A}, α_{1B} and α_{1D}-adrenoceptors, which correspond to the cloned α_{1a}, α_{1b} and α_{1d}-adrenoceptors, respectively, have been described. Although the three cloned subtypes are well characterized, their tissue distribution and function remain to be established.

The proposition that a given adrenoceptor subtype may be responsible for the contractility of prostatic and urethral smooth muscle cells led to the concept that drugs selective for this subtype may exhibit functional uroselectivity [7]. In the human prostate, the three cloned subtypes have been identified and the $\alpha_{1a/A}$-adrenoceptor subtype has been described to be the most abundant receptor subtype in prostatic smooth muscle [8, 9]. Comparison of the affinities of several α_1-adrenoceptor antagonists to the cloned α_1-adrenoceptor subtypes revealed that only few show selectivity for the $\alpha_{1a/A}$-adrenoceptor subtype, whereas most of them had a similar affinity for the three subtypes (table 1).

The α_{1a}-adrenoceptor has been identified in the prostatic tissue using various techniques, but its functional role remains controversial despite the fact that its involvement in mediating prostatic smooth muscle contractility has been extensively investigated [10–12]. Attempts to evaluate the relationship between the selectivity for the α_{1a}-adrenoceptor subtype and functional in vitro selectivity for the urinary tract challenged the relevance of the selectivity for the $\alpha_{1a/A}$-adrenoceptor subtype in predicting functional uroselectivity [13–16]. The conclusions depend upon the compounds evaluated, the origin of receptors used to estimate affinities (cloned vs. native, human vs. animal) and the way functional selectivity was assessed. In the rabbit urethra, in vitro, the α_{1a}-adrenoceptor antagonists tamsulosin, 5-Me-urapidil and WB4101, but not RS-17053, produced a parallel rightward shift of the phenylephrine dose-response curve, indicative of competitive antagonism [16]. Thus, RS-17053, which, among the compounds tested, showed high selectivity for the α_{1a}-adrenoceptor subtype (table 1), did not shift the phenylephrine dose-response curve. In addition, when the affinity values for the human cloned α_{1a}-adrenoceptor subtype of a variety of α_1-adrenoceptor antagonists (pKi) [13, 17, 18] were compared with their efficacy in antagonizing phenylephrine-contracted rabbit urethra strips (pK_B) [15,

Table 2. Affinity of various α_1-adrenoceptor antagonists for the cloned α_{1a}-adrenoceptor (pK_i), potency to relax rabbit urethra contracted with phenylephrine (pK_B or pA_2) and their ratios of affinity over potency, expressed by the negative log of the difference between pK_i and pK_B (pA_2)

Compounds	Affinities for human cloned α_{1a}-adrenoceptors (pK_i)	Potencies in the rabbit urethra (pK_B/pA_2)	Ratios affinity/potency
Tamsulosin	9.70 [20]	8.85 [16]	7
Prazosin	9.70 [17]	7.71 [16]	33
WB4101	9.41 [17]	7.95 [16]	29
RS-17053	8.90 [13]	5.86 [16]	1,100
5-Me-urapidil	8.68 [17]	7.70 [16]	10
Alfuzosin	8.20 [17]	6.84 [16]	23
Doxazosin	8.56 [17]	7.50 [15]	11
Terazosin	8.16 [17]	7.10 [16]	11

16], the pK_B values were consistently smaller (by 7- to 1,100-fold) than the pKi values for the α_{1a}-adrenoceptor subtype. This result suggests that the α_1-adrenoceptor mediating urethral contractions does not have all the characteristics of the α_{1a}-adrenoceptor [15, 16] (table 2).

Furthermore, other recent studies suggest that the characteristics of the functional α_1-adrenoceptor subtype in human prostate are not consistent with those of the α_{1a}-adrenoceptor subtype [14, 19]. This functional α_1-adrenoceptor subtype seems to correspond better to a subtype with low affinity for prazosin [20] and which is discriminated by RS-17053 [14]. The data reported with RS-17053 by Ford et al. [14], and further confirmed with additional selective antagonists by Kenny et al. [18] and van der Graaf et al. [16] indicated that cloned α_{1a}-adrenoceptors and the α_1-adrenoceptors mediating contractile responses to norepinephrine in prostatic tissues in vitro were different. The receptor mediating smooth muscle contraction of the urethra seems to have the characteristics of the α_{1L}-adrenoceptor which has been recently described to be functionally involved in the contraction of lower urinary tract tissue [14].

Therefore, data supporting a relationship between selectivity for the $\alpha_{1a/A}$-adrenoceptor subtype and functional uroselectivity are still lacking. Neither the affinity nor the selectivity of the α_1-adrenoceptor antagonists for the $\alpha_{1a/A}$-adrenoceptor subtype allow us to predict their in vitro efficacy in antagonizing the contraction of urethral or prostatic tissues induced by activation of α_1-adrenoceptors.

Is α_1-Adrenoceptor Subtype Selectivity Predictive of Functional Uroselectivity?

In order to measure functional uroselectivity, various models have been developed to allow the assessment of the respective action of α_1-adrenoceptor antagonists on blood and urethral pressures.

One of the first models which was established allowed us to measure the effects of α_1-adrenoceptor antagonists on urethral pressure (UP) in hypertonia induced by hypogastric nerve stimulation in anesthetized cats compared to the effects on blood pressure (BP) in spontaneously hypertensive rats (SHR) [21]. Three α_1-adrenoceptor antagonists were evaluated following oral or intraduodenal administration in this model in which sympathetic tone was physiologically stimulated. The ratio of doses needed to reduce UP in cats over the doses needed to reduce BP in SHR provided an index to compare the relative uroselectivity of the tested drugs. Under these conditions, the uroselectivity index was different for the three α_1-adrenoceptor antagonists, ranking from 11 for alfuzosin to 1 for prazosin.

The functional role of α_1-adrenoceptor subtypes, in the lower urinary tract and cardiovascular system under conditions of pharmacological stimulation by infusion of noradrenaline or phenylephrine, have also been reported in various other comparative in vivo studies with selective α_1-adrenoceptor antagonists.

In anesthetized dogs, urethral and arterial pressures were increased by injection of phenylephrine and the antagonist effects of various α_1-adrenoceptor antagonists tested [13, 22]. Tamsulosin, like doxazosin and prazosin, antagonized the increases in UP and BP with similar potency and therefore, did not show functional uroselectivity, whereas 5-Me-urapidil antagonized the increases in UP more potently than increases in BP. On the other hand, Testa et al. [12] showed that tamsulosin and rec15/2739 inhibited noradrenaline-induced increases in prostatic pressure with a respective selectivity ratio of 10 and 100 over the reduction in basal blood pressure. Accordingly, Shibashaky et al. [23] showed that tamsulosin was more potent in reducing phenylephrine-induced increases in UP than in BP in female dogs. Recently, Brune et al. [24] investigated the effects of tamsulosin, doxazosin and terazosin on phenylephrine-induced increases in UP and BP in conscious dogs and reported weak uroselectivity for tamsulosin at one of the doses tested. The use of agonists with a different selectivity for α-adrenoceptor subtypes (phenylephrine vs. noradrenaline) or end organ responses (prostatic urethra vs. urethra) may account for some of

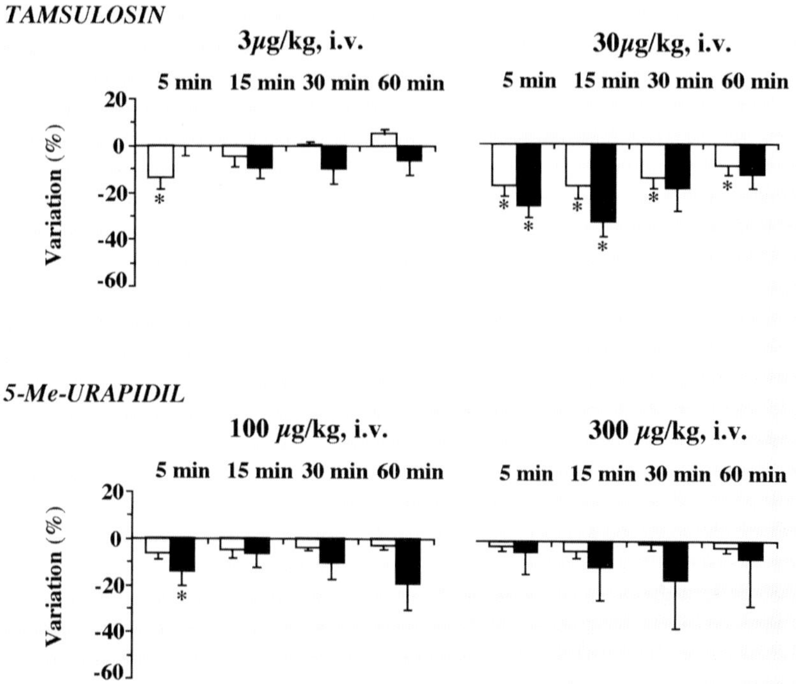

Fig. 1. Effects of selective α_{1a}-adrenoceptor antagonists on UP (■) and BP (□) following intravenous administration in conscious rats [15]. The two doses presented here are the lowest active dose and the highest dose tested. * $p < 0.05$, statistically different from the control group, one-way Anova.

the described discrepancies. In general, however, in the various dog models, the potency to decrease pharmacologically stimulated UP and BP could be correlated with selectivity for the $\alpha_{1a/A}$-adrenoceptor subtype.

In anesthetized cats, doxazosin and terazosin were shown to be active on the sympathetic drive to the bladder and on blood pressure within the same dose range, even though doxazosin induced less tachycardia than terazosin [25].

More recently, uroselectivity was evaluated in conscious male rats by the simultaneous measurement of both BP and UP under normal conditions [26]. Their modification by the administration of α_1-adrenoceptor antagonists was thus evaluated in the absence of exogenous sympathetic stimulation [15]. This model also allowed an evaluation of the potential role of the $\alpha_{1a/A}$-adrenoceptor subtype in functional uroselectivity by using several α_1-adrenoceptor antagonists with different affinities and selectivities for the three α_1-adrenoceptor subtypes. In this study [15], the definition of uroselectivity was based on a reduction in UP without modification in BP (full uroselectivity), a reduction in UP associated with a decrease in BP less than 10% (partial uroselectivity) or a decrease in UP (or no modification of UP) associated with a decrease in BP equal to or greater than 10% (no uroselectivity). Compounds considered to be selective for the $\alpha_{1a/A}$-adrenoceptor, like tamsulosin or 5-Me-urapidil (table 1), did not show functional uroselectivity as decreases in urethral pressure were not achieved in the absence of associated decreases in BP (fig. 1). Conversely, α_1-adrenoceptor antagonists without α_1-adrenoceptor subtype selectivity, like alfuzosin or to a minor extent doxazosin, showed full or partial functional uroselectivity, whereas prazosin and terazosin were not shown to be uroselective (fig. 2). Thus, within the dose range active on UP, these compounds induced variable effects on BP in a manner which was not correlated to their selectivity for the known α_1-adrenoceptor subtypes.

In these studies, the two compounds with the highest affinity for the α_{1a}-adrenoceptor subtype, tamsulosin (pKi = 10.4) and prazosin (pKi = 9.73) were the most potent in affecting BP and the least uroselective. Compounds with higher functional uroselectivity, i.e. alfuzosin and doxazosin have a similar binding profile which is devoid of α_1-adrenoceptor subtype selectivity. Therefore, in this model, functional uroselectivity was not correlated with pharmacological selectivity or affinity for the $\alpha_{1a/A}$-adrenoceptor subtype.

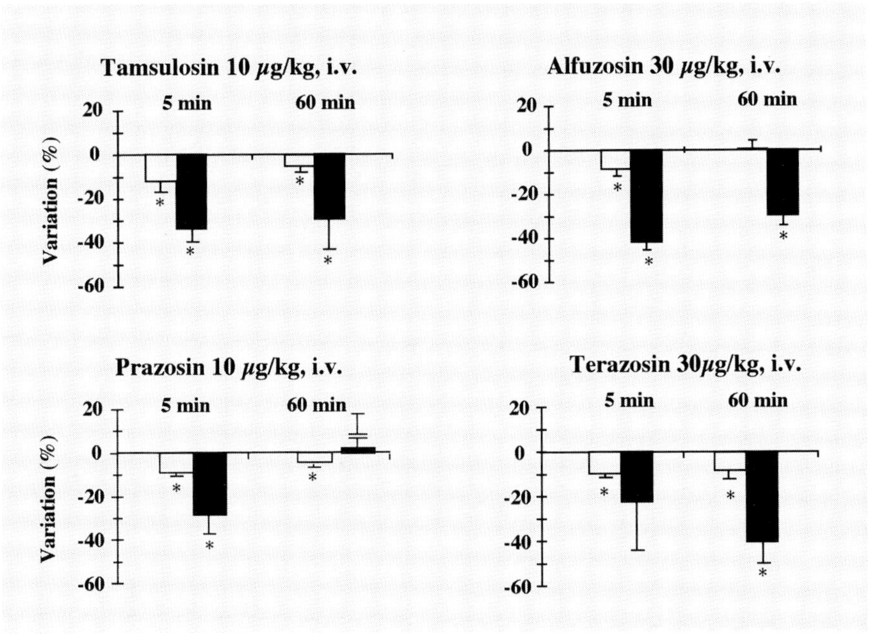

Fig. 2. Comparative uroselectivity of α_1-adrenoceptor antagonists following intravenous administration in conscious rats [15]. The dose presented for each antagonist is the most uroselective dose. ■ = UP; □ = BP. * $p < 0.05$, statistically different from the control group, one-way Anova.

Table 3. Summary of functional uroselectivity for α_1-adrenoceptor antagonists in experimental models

Sympathetic tone	Stimulus	Species	Reference	Results: presence or rank order of uroselectivity	Results: absence of uroselectivity
Physiologically stimulated	sympathetic hyperactivity (genetic)	conscious SHR	21	alfuzosin > terazosin	prazosin
	hypogastric nerve stimulation	anesthetized cat			
Physiological	'normal' sympathetic tone	anesthetized cat	25	–	doxazosin, terazosin
		conscious rat	26	alfuzosin	–
		conscious rat	15	alfuzosin > doxazosin	tamsulosin, prazosin, terazosin, 5-Me-urapidil
Pharmacologically stimulated	phenylephrine	anesthetized dog	13, 22	5-Me urapidil	doxazosin, tamsulosin, prazosin
	phenylephrine	anesthetized dog	23	tamsulosin	
	noradrenaline	anesthetized dog	12	rec15/2739 > tamsulosin	
	phenylephrine	conscious dog	24	tamsulosin	doxazosin, terazosin

In all these studies, with the exception of the latter, α_1-adrenoceptor antagonists were tested against increases in UP and BP induced by agonist injection, electrical stimulation or against a genetically induced hypertension. Studies performed in conscious rats [15, 26] were the first attempt to evaluate the direct effects of α_1-adrenoceptor antagonists in conscious animals under normal adrenergic tone.

Overall, in most of the published studies, under different experimental conditions in which sympathetic tone is maintained by a physiological stimulus, α_1-adrenoceptor antagonists like alfuzosin and to a minor extent doxazosin and terazosin, show functional uroselectivity (table 3), which is not correlated with pharmacological selectivity for the $\alpha_{1a/A}$-adrenoceptor subtype.

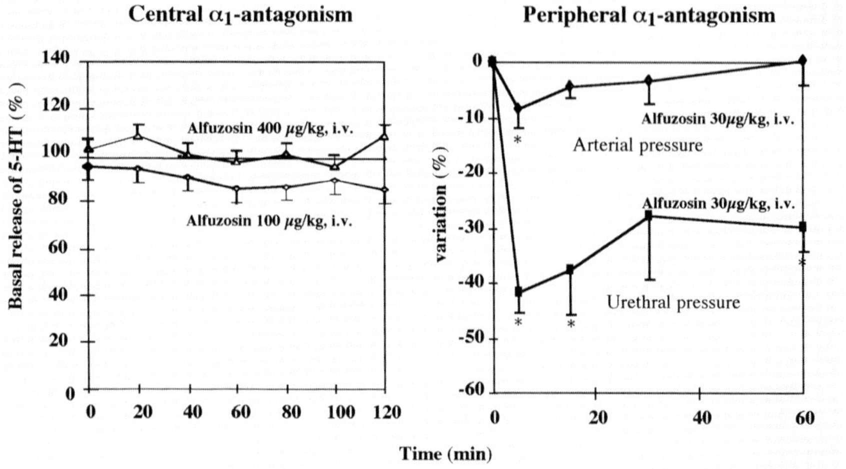

Fig. 3. Comparative central and peripheral α_1-adrenoceptor antagonist activity of alfuzosin [15, 31]. Lack of central α_1-blockade is measured by a normal release of 5-HT following intravenous administration of alfuzosin [31]. Peripheral blockade is measured by the time-course effect of intravenous alfuzosin on BP and UP [15]. * $p < 0.05$, statistically different from the control group, one-way Anova.

Is Brain Penetration an Important Feature for Functional Uroselectivity?

The issue of brain penetration by α_1-adrenoceptor antagonists is of importance since through central action, either beneficial or undesired effects could be expected. It has indeed been proposed that central inhibition of the activity of sympathetic neurones innervating the prostate could improve the efficacy of α_1-adrenoceptor antagonists at the lower urinary tract level [27, 28]. Conversely, several central mechanisms, including those regulating blood pressure, involve central $\alpha_{1a/A}$-adrenoceptors [29, 30]. Blockade of central α_1-adrenoceptors could therefore lead to unwanted side effects.

In the hippocampus, serotonin release is modulated by α_1-adrenoceptor activation and the local measurement of serotonin concentration provides an index of central activity of adrenoceptor antagonists which penetrate the brain. Prazosin, and to a lesser extent terazosin, given intravenously, decrease basal serotonin release in the hippocampus, which is indicative of brain penetration [31]. As shown in figure 3, alfuzosin, at doses 10–40 times higher than those effective on urethral pressure [15], does not modify hippocampal serotonin release [31]. Thus, in the rat, alfuzosin shows functional uroselectivity by decreasing UP at doses which do not modify BP or penetrate the brain. Ramage et al. [25] showed that terazosin and doxazosin had a central inhibitory action on sympathetic drive in anesthetized cats, which could explain their activity at both the lower urinary tract and cardiovascular level. Tamsulosin was also suggested to have central inhibitory sympathetic activity which could play a role in its antitachycardic or bradycardic effects shown in anesthetized rats [32]. From available data, it appears that α_1-adrenoceptor antagonists which can cross the blood-brain barrier have the potential to induce side-effects even though other beneficial effects may be expected at the level of the lower urinary tract.

In conclusion, the presented studies demonstrate that functional uroselectivity of adrenoceptor antagonists cannot be extrapolated from either their receptor affinity or receptor subtype selectivity. In the conscious male rat under normal adrenergic tone, the most uroselective drugs were alfuzosin and, over a more limited dose range, doxazosin while tamsulosin, 5-Me-urapidil, prazosin and terazosin were either partially uroselective or not uroselective. This uroselectivity is therefore not correlated with a selective affinity for the α_{1a}-adrenoceptor subtype.

The actual state of knowledge on α_1-adrenoceptor subtype distribution and function does not support a role of pharmacological uroselectivity in predicting functional uroselectivity. However, functional uroselectivity, measured in animal models, can be achieved in the absence of selectivity for the α_1-adrenoceptor subtypes so far described.

Acknowledgments

The authors wish to thank P. Lluel for his invaluable help in the preparation of the manuscript.

References

1 Lepor H, Shapiro E: Characterization of alpha1-adrenergic receptors in human benign prostatic hyperplasia. J Urol 1987;132:1226–1229.

2 Andersson KE : Pharmacology of the lower urinary tract smooth muscle and penile erectile tissues. Pharmacol Rev 1993;45:253–308.

3 Caine M, Pfau A, Pelberg S: The use of alpha-adrenergic blockers in benign prostatic obstruction. Br J Urol 1976;48:255–263.

4 Cockett ATK, Aso Y, Denis L, Khoury S, Barry M, Carlton CE, et al: Recommendations of the International Consensus Committee concerning: 4. BPH treatment recommendations; in Cockett ATK, et al (eds): The International Consultation on Benign Prostatic Hyperplasia (BPH), Paris, 1991, pp 287–288.

5 Andersson KE: Uroselectivity; in Proceedings of the Third International Consultation on Benign Prostatic Hyperplasia, Monaco, 1995, pp 541–542.

6 Langer SZ: Presynaptic regulation of catecholamine release. Biochem Pharmacol 1974;23: 1793–1799.

7 Chapple CR, Burt RP, Andersson PO, Greengrass P, Wyllie M, Marshall I : Alpha1-adrenoceptor subtypes in the human prostate. Br J Urol 1994;74:585–589.

8 Lepor H, Tang R, Kobayashi S, Shapiro E, Forray C, Wetzel J, Gluchowski C: Localization of the α_{1A}-adrenoceptor in the human prostate. J Urol 1995;154:2096–2099.

9 Taniguchi N, Ukai Y, Tanaka T, Yano J, Kimura K, Morimaya N, Kawabe K : Identification of alpha1-adrenoceptor subtypes in the human prostatic urethra. Naunyn-Schmiedeberg's Arch Pharmacol 1997;355:412–416.

10 Kawabe K: Efficacy and safety of tamsulosin in the treatment of benign prostatic hyperplasia. Br J Urol 1995;76:63–67.

11 Michel MC, Insel PA: Comparison of cloned and pharmacologically defined rat tissue α_1-adrenoceptor subtypes. Naunyn-Schmiedeberg's Arch Pharmacol 1994;350:136–142.

12 Testa R, Sironi G, Colombo D, Greto L, Leonardi A : Rec 15/2739 a new α_1-antagonist selective for the lower urinary tract: In vivo studies. Neuronal Urodyn 1994;13:471–473.

13 Blue DR Jr, Daniels DV, Ford APDW, Williams TJ, Eglen RM, Clarke DE : Pharmacological assessment of the α_1-adrenoceptor (α_1-AR) antagonist tamsulosin (abstract 737). J Urol 1997;157:190.

14 Ford APDW, Arredondo NF, Blue DR Jr, Bonhaus DW, Jasper J, Kava MS, Lesnik J, Pfister JR, Shieh IA, Vimont RL, Williams TJ, Mcneal JE, Stamey TA, Clarke DE: RS-17053 (N-[2-(2-cyclopropylmethoxyphenoxy) ethyl]-5-chloro-α,α-dimethyl-1-H-indole-3-ethanamine hydrochloride), a selective α_1-adrenoceptor antagonist, displays low affinity for functional α_1-adrenoceptors in human prostate: Implications for adrenoceptor classification. Eur J Pharmacol 1996;49:209–215.

15 Martin DJ, Lluel P, Guillot E, Coste A, Jammes D, Angel I: Comparative alpha1-adrenoceptor subtype selectivity and functional uroselectivity of alpha1-adrenoceptor antagonists. J Pharmacol Exp Ther 1997;282:228–235.

16 Van Der Graaf PH, Deplanne V, Duquenne C, Angel I: Analysis of α_1-adrenoceptors in rabbit lower urinary tract and mesenteric artery. Eur J Pharmacol 1997;327:25–32.

17 Forray C, Bard JA, Wetzel JM, Chiu G, Shapiro E, Tang R, Lepor H, Hartig PR, Weinshank RL, Branchek TA, Gluchowsi C: The alpha1-adrenoceptor that mediates smooth muscle contraction in human prostate has the pharmacological properties of the cloned alpha-1c subtype. Mol Pharmacol 1994;45:703–708.

18 Kenny BA, Miller AM, Williamson IJR, O'Connell J, Chalmers DH, Naylor AM: Evaluation of the pharmacological selectivity profile of α_1 adrenoceptors: Binding, functional and in vivo studies. Br J Pharmacol 1996;118:871–878.

19 Testa R, Guarneri L, Taddei C, Poggesi E, Angelico P, Sartani A, Leonardi A, Gofrit ON, Meretyk S, Caine M: Functional antagonistic activity of rec15/2739, a novel alpha-1 antagonist selective for the lower urinary tract, on noradrenaline-induced contraction of human prostate and mesenteric artery. J Pharmacol Exp Ther 1996;277:1237–1246.

20 Muramatsu I, Oshita M, Ohmura T, Kigoshi S, Akino H, Gobara M, Okada K: Pharmacological characterization of α_1-adrenoceptor subtypes in the human prostate: Functional and binding studies. Br J Urol 1994;74:572–578.

21 Lefèvre-Borg F, Lechaire J, O'Connor S: In vivo uroselectivity of alfuzosin compared to prazosin and terazosin. Br J Pharmacol 1992; 106:84P.

22 Kenny BA, Naylor AM, Carter AJ, Read AM, Greengrass PM, Wyllie MG: Effect of alpha-1-adrenoceptor antagonists on prostatic pressure and blood pressure in the anaesthetised dog. Urology 1994;44:52–57.

23 Shibasaki M, Sudoh K, Inagaki O, Uchida W, Honda K: Effect of the optical isomers of YM-12617 on increased intra-urethral pressure induced by phenylephrine in anaesthetised dogs. J Auton Pharmacol 1992;12:263–268.

24 Brune ME, Katwala SP, Milicic I, Hancock AA, Kerwin JF Jr: Simultaneous evaluation of the effects of alpha1-adrenergic antagonists on vascular and prostatic smooth muscle in intact conscious dogs. J Urol 1996;155:332A.

25 Ramage AG, Wyllie MG : A comparison of the effects of doxazosin and terazosin on the spontaneous sympathetic drive to the bladder and related organs in anaesthetized cats. Eur J Pharmacol 1995;294:645–650.

26 Martin D, Jammes D, Angel I: Effects of Alfuzosin on urethral and blood pressures in conscious male rats. Life Sci 1995;57:PL387–391.

27 Danuser H, Thor KB: Inhibition of central sympathetic and somatic outflow to the lower urinary tract of the cat by the α_1-adrenergic receptor antagonist prazosin. J Urol 1995;153: 1308–1312.

28 Andersson KE: Alpha1-adrenergic receptor blockade in the male lower urinary tract and other body systems. Scand J Urol Nephrol 1995;29:13–20.

29 Baum T, Shropshire AT: Central and peripheral contribution to the antihypertensive action of indoramin. Eur J Pharmacol 1975;32:30–38.

30 Ramage AG: Evidence for a central sympathoinhibitory action of prazosin and indoramin. Eur J Pharmacol 1986;121:83–89.

31 Rouquier L, Claustre Y, Benavides J : α_1-Adrenoceptor antagonists differentially control serotonin release in the hippocampus and striatum: A microdialysis study. Eur J Pharmacol 1994;261:59–64.

32 Yoshioka M, Togashi H, Abe M, Ikeda T, Matsumoto M, Saito H: Central sympathoinhibitory action of a new type of alpha-1 adrenoceptor antagonist, YM-617, in rats. J Pharmacol Exp Ther 1990;253:427–431.

33 Chess-Williams R, Chaple CR, Verfuth F, Noble AJ, Couldwell C, Michel MC: The effects of SB 216469, an antagonist which discriminates between the α_{1A}-adrenoceptor and the human prostatic α_1-adrenoceptor. Br J Pharmacol 1996;119:1093–1100.

European Urology

Eur Urol 1998;33(suppl 2):19–27

Roger S. Kirby

Department of Urology, St. George's Hospital, London, UK

Clinical Uroselectivity of Alfuzosin in the Treatment of Benign Prostatic Hyperplasia

Key Words
α-Blocker
Benign prostatic hyperplasia
Alfuzosin
Uroselectivity

Abstract

The efficacy of alfuzosin in improving lower urinary tract symptoms and relieving bladder outlet obstruction has been demonstrated in numerous short- and long-term placebo-controlled studies and large-scale open studies, involving over 16,000 patients with symptomatic benign prostatic hyperplasia (BPH). Treatment with sustained release alfuzosin (5 mg twice daily) for 3 months resulted in a 5-point reduction in the International Prostate Symptom Score and a 29% increase in urinary flow rate. The benefits of alfuzosin have been confirmed in general practice. A 1-year prospective study of 5,849 men with clinical BPH treated with alfuzosin showed a 51% reduction in mean total symptom score, with a 56% decrease in mean irritative symptoms. Improvement in health-related quality of life of 3 years' duration have been recorded, including a reduction in the frequency of both diurnal and nocturnal micturition. Alfuzosin has a good safety profile. Unlike most other α_1-blockers, a low risk of first-dose effect is seen, conveniently eliminating the necessity of dose titration at initiation of therapy. Postural symptoms related to orthostatic hypotension (a common side-effect of α_1-blockers) are infrequent, including in the elderly and hypertensives. Central nervous system effects are also limited due to poor penetration of the blood-brain barrier. In conclusion, the positive benefits/risk ratio of alfuzosin allows it to be classified as a uroselective α_1-blocker, which provides a beneficial contribution to the management of symptomatic BPH.

Introduction

Currently, the two main classes of pharmacological therapy for clinical benign prostatic hyperplasia (BPH) are α_1-blockers and 5α-reductase inhibitors. The latter is a hormone-related approach aimed at reducing prostate size by lowering the level of dihydrotestosterone. The only drug approved in this class is finasteride. In contrast, α_1-blockers act by reducing prostate and urethral muscle tone. Unlike the 5α-reductase inhibitors, α_1-blockers have an early onset of action, with evidence of efficacy within 1–2 weeks [1].

The application of α_1-blockers for the relief of bladder outlet obstruction due to BPH was first proposed by Caine et al. [2] 1976. By antagonizing the effect of noradrenaline at the α_1-adrenoceptor, α_1-blockers reduce smooth muscle cell tone in the bladder neck, prostatic urethra, prostate capsule and prostatic adenoma [2, 3]. The consequence of this is a reduction in the dynamic component of bladder outlet obstruction. α_1-Blockers have also

KARGER

Fax + 41 61 306 12 34
E-Mail karger@karger.ch
www.karger.com

0302–2838/98/0338–0019$15.00/0

This article is also accessible online at:
http://BioMedNet.com/karger

Roger S. Kirby
149 Harley Street
London W1N 2DE (UK)
Tel. +44 171 935 97 20, Fax +44 171 224 57 06

been shown to reduce the irritative (storage, i.e. urgency, nocturia, daytime frequency) symptoms of BPH.

The side-effects produced by α_1-blockers (e.g. orthostatic hypotension, dizziness and headache) can be substantial in certain patient groups, and may be attributed to non-prostatic α_1-adrenoceptor blockade. For this reason, attempts have been made to identify α_1-blockers that have a selective effect on the prostate. The concept of uroselectivity of α_1-blockers has been developed in order to identify agents with the best ratio between benefits on BPH symptoms and the incidence of potentially bothersome side-effects. Clinical uroselectivity was defined by Dr. Karl-Eric Andersson at the International Consultation on Benign Prostatic Hyperplasia, held in Monaco in 1995 as: 'desired effects on obstruction and lower urinary tract symptoms (LUTS) related to adverse effects' [4].

Alfuzosin, a quinazoline derivative, is a selective and competitive α_1-adrenoceptor antagonist. It has been shown to reduce urethral pressure and resistance, bladder outlet resistance, bladder instability and symptoms associated with BPH. Alfuzosin has been approved in France for the treatment of symptomatic BPH since 1988 and subsequently in numerous other European countries.

Benefits of α_1-Blocker Therapy for BPH

Infravesical obstruction in men with BPH is composed of two components: (1) a dynamic component related to the tone of smooth muscle fibres in the bladder neck, surgical capsule and fibromuscular stroma, and (2) an anatomical or static component represented by the physical presence of the hyperplastic tissue itself [5]. Shapiro et al. [6] have shown that 39% of the total prostate volume in men with BPH consists of smooth muscle fibres. Attempts to quantify the dynamic and static contribution of obstruction in BPH have concluded that around 40% of the total urethral pressure is due to α-adrenergic tone [7]. The use of α_1-blockers to reduce adrenergic tone has translated into clinical benefits. Results indicate an approximate 30% increase in urinary flow rates, with a corresponding improvement in LUTS [8], as well as a 29% reduction in residual urine volume [9].

To provide optimal benefit, the α_1-blocker should exert maximum effect on the prostate and the bladder, bringing about an improvement in urinary flow rate and LUTS. At the same time, its effects on the cardiovascular and central nervous systems should be minimal, resulting in few concomitant adverse effects.

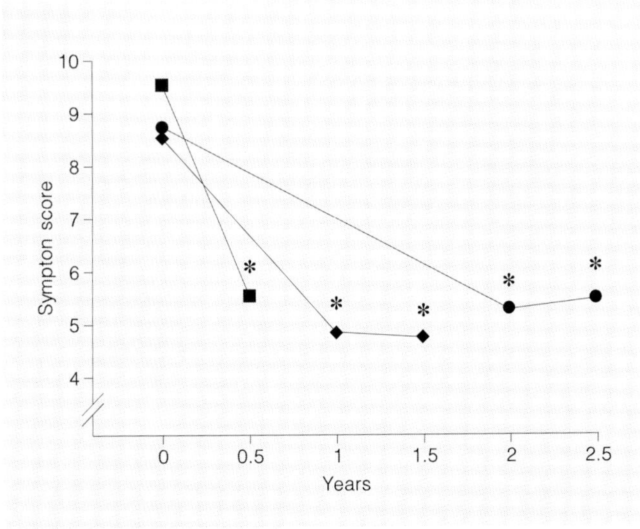

Fig. 1. Long-term maintenance of symptomatic improvement with alfuzosin [12]. ■ = 6-month placebo-controlled study (n = 251); ◆ = 1-year open extension (n = 131); ● = 2-year open extension (n = 50). * $p < 0.001$.

Efficacy of Alfuzosin

The efficacy of alfuzosin in improving LUTS has been demonstrated in 11 placebo-controlled trials involving over 16,000 patients with symptomatic BPH. A placebo-controlled study by Jardin et al. [10] conducted in 518 patients with BPH over a 6-month period, showed that alfuzosin significantly improved obstructive and irritative symptoms ($p = 0.0004$ for total Boyarsky score), urinary flow rates ($p < 0.05$ for mean flow rates at 6 months) and decreased the residual urine volume ($p = 0.017$) in comparison with placebo. Moreover, alfuzosin was shown to reduce the incidence of acute urinary retention compared with placebo (0.4% vs. 2.6%, respectively; $p = 0.04$).

As moderately symptomatic patients can benefit from long-term drug therapy, this 6-month controlled study was continued on an open basis for a further 12 months [11]. Of 122 patients completing 12 months therapy, all obstructive and irritative symptoms were improved; the Boyarsky score decreased from 8.7 ± 0.3 at baseline to 5.2 ± 0.3 at 24 months [12]. Urinary flow rates also improved with peak flow rate increasing from 13.6 ml/s at baseline to 14.6 ml/s after 18 months [11]. Long-term maintenance of symptomatic improvement up to 30 months was demonstrated in a further open extension of this study involving 50 patients [12] (fig. 1).

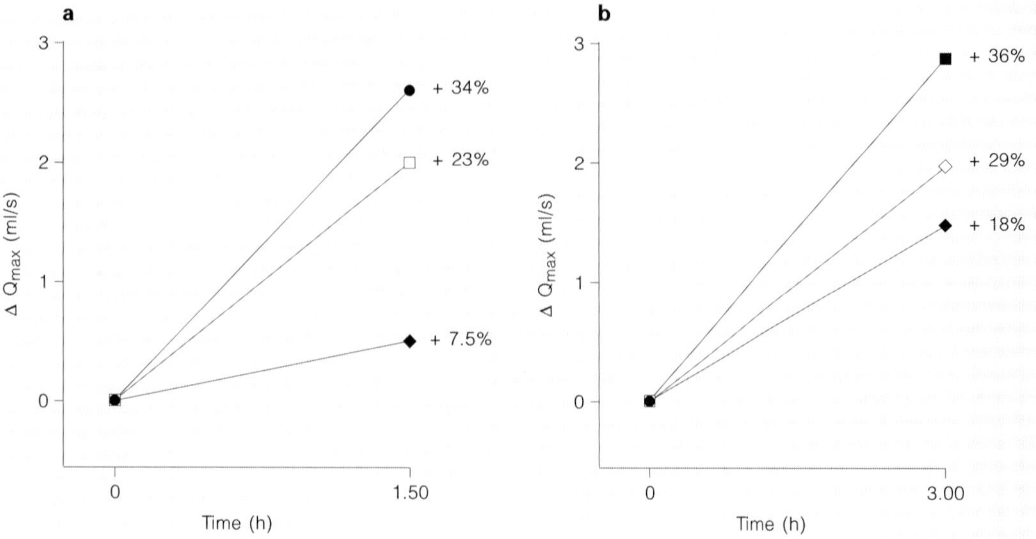

Fig. 2. Effect of first-dose alfuzosin on maximum urinary flow rate (Q_{max}). **a** IR formulation. □ = Alfuzosin, 1.25 mg (n = 31); ● = Alfuzosin, 2.5 mg (n = 31); ◆ = Placebo (n = 31). **b** SR formulation. ◇ = Alfuzosin, 3 mg (n = 57); ■ = Alfuzosin, 5 mg (n = 57); ◆ = Placebo (n = 59).

The magnitude of the improvement in LUTS observed in clinical trials has been confirmed in general practice. In a 1-year prospective study, 5,849 men with clinical BPH were treated with alfuzosin by general practitioners [13]. A reduction in mean total symptom score of 51% was recorded; the mean irritative symptom score was decreased by 56%. Irritative symptoms are of particular clinical interest, as urgency and nocturia are perceived by patients as the most bothersome symptoms in their daily lives. This study also confirmed that the efficacy was maximum from the third month of treatment and that it was unrelated to prostate size and initial residual urine volume. In addition, only 0.3% of patients developed acute urinary retention, which is consistent with the 0.4% incidence observed in a 6-month controlled study [10]. The level of improvement observed was maintained at 2 years in a cohort of 4,591 patients who continued treatment [14].

Alfuzosin has been shown to improve maximum urinary flow rates (Q_{max}) from the first dose in two placebo-controlled studies [15, 16]. Dose-dependent increases in Q_{max} at peak plasma concentration (90 min for the immediate release [IR] formulation; 180 min for the SR formulation) were observed (fig. 2). A 34% increase in Q_{max} was recorded after administration of 2.5 mg IR alfuzosin and a 36% increase after 5 mg SR alfuzosin.

Optimization of the Therapeutic Benefit of Alfuzosin

An SR formulation for twice-daily administration of alfuzosin has been developed to enhance patient compliance compared with IR alfuzosin, which has to be given three times daily. In fact, once-daily and twice-daily regimens have been shown to be associated with significantly better compliance (73 and 70%, respectively) than three-times daily regimens (52%) [17]. The efficacy of this new formulation has been confirmed in a placebo-controlled trial involving 390 patients with BPH treated for 12 weeks [18]. A 5-point (31%) decrease in the International Prostate Symptom Score (IPSS) was recorded after 3 months treatment with alfuzosin compared with a 3.4 point (18%) decrease in the placebo group ($p = 0.007$); improvement in symptom score with alfuzosin was significantly ($p < 0.001$) better than placebo after 1 month (fig. 3). In patients with an IPSS score ≥13 at inclusion, the improvement in IPSS was 6.7 (36%) and 4.0 (22%) in the alfuzosin and placebo groups, respectively ($p = 0.002$). Q_{max} was also improved by 29% after 3 months, the difference between alfuzosin and placebo being significant from the first month until the end of the study ($p = 0.0004$) (fig. 4).

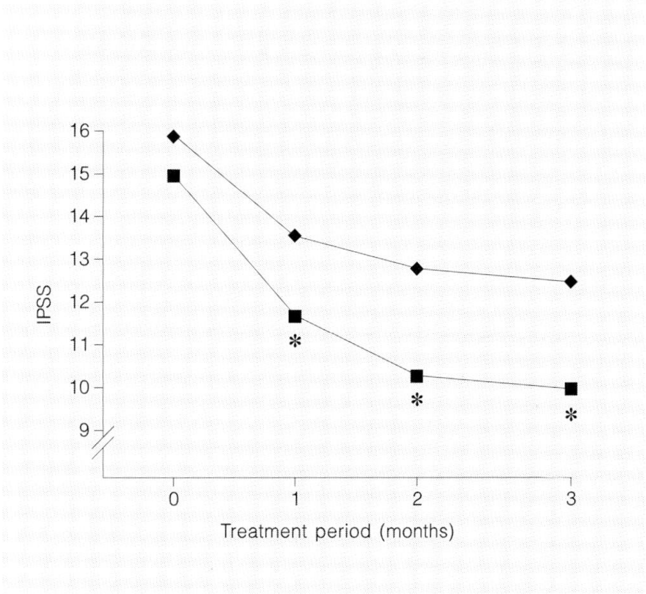

Fig. 3. Effect of sustained release alfuzosin, 5 mg twice daily (n = 191; ■) on LUTS. ◆ = Placebo (n = 191). *p = 0.003. Adapted from Buzelin et al. [18].

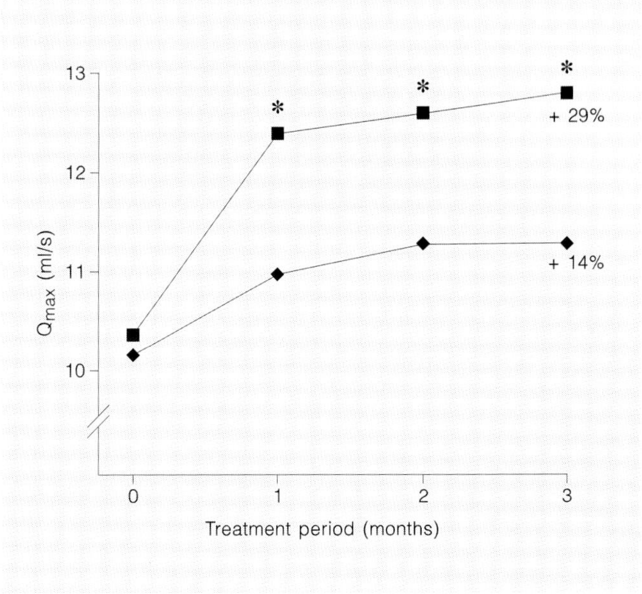

Fig. 4. Effect of SR alfuzosin, 5 mg twice daily (n = 167; ■) on maximum urinary flow rate (Q_{max}). ◆ = Placebo (n = 163). p = 0.0004. Adapted from Buzelin et al. [18].

Comparative Efficacy of Alfuzosin

The efficacy of alfuzosin in relieving BPH symptoms and improving flow rates has been shown to be comparable to several other α_1-blockers. A study by Buzelin et al. [19] compared 3 weeks treatment with alfuzosin, 2.5 mg three times daily, and prazosin, 2 mg twice daily, in 103 patients with BPH [19]. Voiding symptoms, assessed on the basis of the Boyarsky Symptom Score, were significantly ($p < 0.001$) improved in both groups (alfuzosin –2.6; prazosin –2.8). Q_{max} increased similarly with alfuzosin (2.6 ± 0.6 ml/s) and prazosin (2.9 ± 0.7 ml/s). In addition, alfuzosin (immediate release), 7.5 mg/day, was shown to be as effective as tamsulosin, 0.4 mg/day, in improving symptoms and flow rates when both drugs were administered for 12 weeks [20].

Placebo-controlled studies on doxazosin [21] and terazosin [22] indicate improvements in symptoms and urinary flow rate comparable to those recorded with alfuzosin. A 16-week study of doxazosin in 100 patients with BPH resulted in a mean symptom score (AUA) improvement of 5.7 points (40.1%) compared with a 2.5 point (16%) reduction in the placebo group. Q_{max} was improved by 29.9% vs. 7.1% in the doxazosin and placebo groups, respectively. A 1-year prospective study on terazosin in 1,949 patients resulted in symptom score improvements of 7.6 (37.8%) and 3.7 (18.4%) points in the terazosin and placebo groups, respectively. With regard to improvement in Q_{max}, increases of 2.2 ml/s vs. 0.8 ml/s were recorded in the terazosin and placebo groups (data on 277 patients).

Risks Associated with α_1-Blockers

BPH is a common condition in older men: approximately 50% of men over the age of 50 will show histological signs of the disease, with the incidence rising to 88% in men aged 80 years [23]. Although BPH can have a significant impact on the quality of life of sufferers [24], it should be noted that it is seldom a life-threatening disease and, as such, drugs used to treat the condition need to be well tolerated. As observed by the Alpha Blocker Committee of the Third International Consultation on BPH, α_1-blockers have demonstrated quality of life improvement and acceptable safety to be considered an appropriate treatment option in patients with bothersome symptoms of BPH.

Potential adverse events with α_1-blockers relate mainly to their effects on the cardiovascular system, e.g. dizziness, headache, palpitations/tachycardia, postural hypotension and syncope, or to blood-brain barrier penetra-

Table 1. Safety profile of terazosin up to 10 mg once daily, administered for 1 year, alone or in combination with finasteride 5 mg once daily, in the Veterans' Administration Cooperative Study (adapted from Lepor et al. [25])

Adverse events	Placebo (n = 305)	Finasteride (n = 310)	Terazosin (n = 305)	Combination (n = 309)	p[1]
Dizziness, %	7	8	26	21	<0.001
Asthenia, %	7	7	14	14	0.002
Impotence, %	5	9	6	9	0.05
Ejaculatory abnormality, %	1	2	0.3	7	<0.001
Decreased libido, %	1	5	3	5	0.05
Syncope, %	0	1	1	2	0.20
Postural hypotension, %	1	2	8	9	<0.001

[1] p relates to overall difference among the 4 groups.

tion, leading to central events such as asthenia and somnolence. The main serious side-effects associated with α_1-blockers are postural symptoms relative to orthostatic hypotension. These rare events are a particular concern in the elderly BPH population as they can result in severe morbidity from associated falls. The risks involved with the use of α_1-blockers have been demonstrated in the Veterans Administration Cooperative Study, which compared the efficacy and safety of terazosin, finasteride and their combination with placebo over a 1-year period [25]. Postural hypotension was shown to be four times more frequent in patients who received terazosin than in those who received placebo or finasteride; dizziness was three times more frequent and asthenia twice as frequent (table 1). As far as dizziness, hypotension and asthenia are concerned, doxazosin has a similar adverse event profile as terazosin, as indicated in two placebo-controlled studies (table 2) [26, 27], where similar figures were observed.

Table 2. Commonly reported adverse events with doxazosin (adapted from Roehrborn et al. [26] and Fawzy et al. [27])

Adverse events	Roehrborn et al. [26][1]		Fawzy et al. [27][2]	
	placebo (n = 143)	doxazosin (n = 196)	placebo (n = 50)	doxazosin (n = 50)
Dizziness, %	6.3	17.3	4	24
Headache, %	9.8	10.7	4	12
Fatigue, %	2.8	10.7	4	12
Somnolence, %	1.4	5.1	4	10
Hypotension, %	–	4.1	0	8

[1] Doses: 4–12 mg.
[2] Doses: up to 8 mg.

Risk Factors for Orthostatic Blood Pressure Changes

Risk factors for orthostatic blood pressure changes with α_1-blockers can be drug related, linked to the intrinsic properties of the drug, e.g. lack of functional selectivity, but also to its pharmacokinetic profile in humans. After the first administration of an α_1-blocker, symptomatic postural hypotension can occur, which rapidly subsides with protracted treatment. High initial doses and rapid increases in the dose are well known risk factors for this effect, known as the first-dose effect [28]. Consequently, drugs with a significant risk of orthostatic blood pressure changes, such as prazosin, need to be prescribed with an initial titration. Caution is also needed with terazosin and doxazosin.

Another risk factor related to the drug is its rapid uptake and studies indicate that this can be reduced with modified release formulations. A study of tamsulosin in healthy volunteers showed that higher doses of a modified release formulation could be given without increasing the incidence of orthostatic hypotension recorded with lower doses of an IR formulation [29]. The risk of orthostatic blood pressure changes with α_1-blockers can also be related to certain patient groups. Well known risk factors include ageing, associated hypertension and related treatment with antihypertensives, and plasma volume depletion [30, 31].

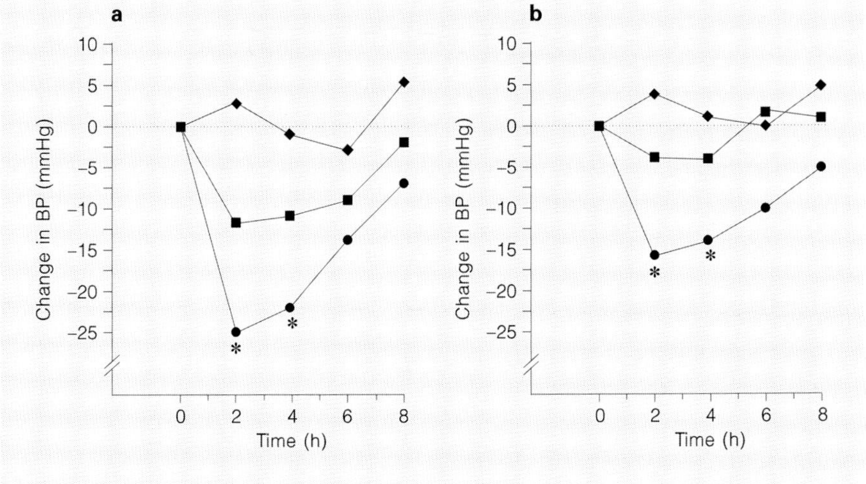

Fig. 5. Comparison of the effect of a first dose of IR alfuzosin, 5 mg (■) and prazosin, 1 mg (●), on orthostatic changes in blood pressure (BP) in healthy volunteers (n = 6). * $p < 0.05$ vs. baseline and placebo (◆). Adapted from Scott et al. [36]. **a** Systolic blood pressure. **b** Diastolic blood pressure.

Safety Profile of Alfuzosin

The safety profile of alfuzosin has been defined by numerous clinical studies conducted with both the IR and the SR formulations, from surveys of patients treated by general practitioners and from large post-marketing surveillance data collected in European countries since its first launch in 1988. In total, experience relates to over 300 million days of treatment.

The two main reasons for the good safety profile of alfuzosin relate to its functional uroselectivity and to its low blood-brain barrier penetration. The functional selectivity of an α_1-blocker indicates a preferential effect on urethral pressure without significant effects on either the cardiovascular or central nervous systems. Various models have been developed to compare the respective action of α_1-blockers on blood and urethral pressures. One method is to measure the effects on urethral hypertonia induced by hypogastric nerve stimulation in anaesthetized cats and the effects on blood pressure in spontaneously hypertensive rats. The ratio of doses needed to reduce urethral pressure by 50% in cats over the dose needed to reduce blood pressure by 20% in rats provides a means of comparing the relative uroselectivity index between drugs. A study by Lefèvre-Borg et al. [32] compared the tissue selectivities of prazosin, terazosin and alfuzosin using this method, and found that alfuzosin demonstrated greater functional uroselectivity than either of the other drugs.

Recently, the effects of alfuzosin on urethral and arterial blood pressure in the same conscious animal (rat) were simultaneously recorded to directly assess its functional uroselectivity in the absence of increased adrenergic tone of external origin. A study by Martin and associates showed that alfuzosin dose-dependently and selectively decreased urethral pressure. A comparative study on alfuzosin, prazosin and tamsulosin, using the same animal model confirmed the preferential effect that alfuzosin has on urethral pressure [34].

The potential for α_1-adrenoceptor antagonists to cross the blood-brain barrier has also been evaluated in animal models. A study by Rouquier et al. [35] showed that, when given by the intravenous route, prazosin, and to a lesser extent terazosin, decrease the α_1-adrenoceptor-mediated release of basal serotonin in the hippocampus. Conversely, alfuzosin did not modify serotonin release, indicating the lack of central α_1-adrenoceptor blockade by the compound and suggesting its restricted penetration of the blood-brain barrier.

Blood Pressure Effects

Alfuzosin has a low risk of first-dose effect. A placebo-controlled, comparative study on prazosin, 1 mg (in BPH therapy, usual intake in a single dose is 2 mg), and IR alfuzosin, 5 mg (usual intake in a single dose is 2.5 mg), was conducted in healthy volunteers to examine this effect [36]. Rapid decreases in standing systolic and diastolic blood pressures were recorded following the first dose of prazosin compared with placebo (fig. 5). In comparison, alfuzosin induced only minor and transient decreases in

Table 3. Overall incidence of adverse events with SR alfuzosin 10 mg/day (adapted from Buzelin et al. [37])

	Placebo (n = 296)	Alfuzosin (n = 292)
Percentage of patients		
With at least one adverse event	15.8	18.5
Withdrawn for an adverse event	5.7	3.4
With an adverse event related to vasodilatation	2.7	2.7
Percentages of most relevant adverse events		
Dizziness	1.3	2.1
Headache	0.7	0.3
Syncope/malaise	–	0.7
Palpitations	1	–
Peripheral oedema	–	0.3
Asthenia	–	0.3

standing systolic blood pressure. The low risk of first-dose effect with alfuzosin means that initial dose titration is not necessary.

The effect of alfuzosin on supine blood pressure was studied in a pooled analysis of two placebo-controlled trials involving 588 patients with BPH [37]. Included in the study were patients at-risk for blood pressure changes, i.e. elderly (51% of patients) and hypertensives (29% of patients). The latter group was defined as patients with treated hypertension and/or systolic blood pressure ≥160 mm Hg and/or diastolic blood pressure ≥100 mm Hg at preinclusion and inclusion visits. Results showed that supine blood pressure changes in the whole population during the first month of treatment were minimal and not clinically relevant. In addition, in hypertensive patients no clinically relevant changes in supine blood pressure with alfuzosin were recorded.

Symptomatic blood pressure changes in orthostatism have been studied during the first month of treatment with SR alfuzosin, as the risk for this side-effect is greatest during this period [37]. Results from the pooled analysis of two-placebo-controlled trials showed that the overall incidence of asymptomatic orthostatic hypotension was slightly more frequent with alfuzosin than with placebo, but that the difference was not statistically significant. The incidence of asymptomatic orthostatic hypotension was higher in the elderly and/or hypertensives, but this did not have any objective consequences on the incidence of adverse events in these subgroups of patients.

Adverse Event Profile of Alfuzosin

The IR formulation of alfuzosin has been shown to be well tolerated in clinical studies. A placebo-controlled study of alfuzosin, 7.5–10 mg/day in three doses, in 518 patients with BPH resulted in a similar overall incidence of adverse events in the placebo and alfuzosin groups. The most common events recorded were dizziness (7.2% and 5.2% in the alfuzosin and placebo groups, respectively) and headache (6.4% and 4.9% in the alfuzosin and placebo groups, respectively) [10]. The incidence of drop-outs due to adverse events was also similar (alfuzosin: 10.8%; placebo: 9.0%).

These results have been confirmed in a French general practice study involving an assessment of 13,389 patients with BPH treated with alfuzosin, 2.5 mg three times daily, for 3 months [38]. In this study of the largest safety data base reported with an α_1-blocker in the treatment of BPH, 3.7% of patients overall discontinued therapy due to adverse events, two-thirds of which were vasodilatory effects, mainly vertigo/dizziness (1.4%), malaise (0.6%), hypotension (0.4%) and headache (0.4%). Three-quarters of all adverse events occurred during the first week of therapy and less than 0.3% of patients reported a first-dose effect.

The adverse event profile of IR alfuzosin, 7.5–10 mg/day, has also been compared to prazosin, 4 mg/day in two short-term, placebo-controlled studies in BPH patients [19, 39]. In a combined analysis of the two studies, vertigo/dizziness was reported in 6 patients in the alfuzosin group (n = 84) compared with 11 in the prazosin group (n = 91); the incidence of syncope/malaise was 1 and 5, respectively, and headache 3 and 9, respectively.

These results suggest that alfuzosin is better tolerated than prazosin in the treatment of BPH. An improved adverse event profile for alfuzosin has resulted from the use of an SR formulation. This has been shown in a pooled analysis [37] of two-placebo-controlled studies of 588 patients treated with SR alfuzosin, 10 mg/day for 1 month [40] or 3 months [18] (table 3). SR alfuzosin was very well tolerated with an overall incidence of adverse events similar to that of placebo (18.5% and 15.8%, respectively) and an overall incidence of drop-out for adverse events lower than that of placebo (3.4% and 5.8%, respectively). Interestingly, the frequency of adverse events related to vasodilatory properties was similar in both groups; the incidence of these events was slightly more frequent during the first month of treatment. A low incidence of asthenia was recorded for alfuzosin. An analysis of subgroup populations of at-risk patients (elderly and/or hypertensives) showed a similar incidence of symptoms potentially related to vasodilation in the alfuzosin and placebo groups during the first month of treatment. The incidence of these symptoms for the different patient categories in the placebo and alfuzosin groups, respectively, was as follows:

- All patients: 2.1% and 1.0%
- ≥65 years: 1.3% and 1.3%
- Hypertensives: 1% and 1%

Comparison with Other α_1-Blockers

Accurate estimates of the comparative incidence of side-effects of various α_1-blockers can only be provided by published direct comparative studies.

Alfuzosin (IR formulation administered in 3 divided doses) was directly compared with prazosin and tamsulosin. Two studies have shown that alfuzosin was better tolerated than prazosin [18, 38]. In a recent study comparing alfuzosin 2.5 mg three times daily and tamsulosin 0.4 mg once daily, both drugs were shown to be well tolerated in patients with BPH. The incidence of overall adverse events, withdrawals for adverse events and postural hypotension with alfuzosin was 48%, 4% and 1% compared with 53%, 8% and 3%, respectively, for tamsulosin [20]. No direct comparative study versus SR alfuzosin has been reported. Nevertheless, its safety profile can be approximately compared to that of various α_1-blockers [41–43] by calculating the ratio of the incidence of withdrawals due to adverse events (% patients) between the drug and placebo. This method provides a ratio lower than 1 only for SR alfuzosin.

Conclusions

The efficacy of alfuzosin in improving symptoms and urodynamic parameters in patients with BPH has been demonstrated in a number of placebo-controlled studies. Positive urodynamic benefits are evident from the first dose, allowing rapid symptom relief. In addition, symptomatic improvement is gained from the first month of therapy and can be maintained for up to 3 years. Alfuzosin has a good safety profile with a low risk of first-dose effect. There is a low incidence of cardiovascular effects such as postural hypotension, even in at-risk groups, as well as a low incidence of CNS effects, such as asthenia, fatigue and somnolence. The large clinical experience from cohorts of patients treated in general practice has confirmed the beneficial results obtained in controlled studies. For patients suffering from BPH, the benefits are emphasized by a progressive improvement in the perceived quality of life. In conclusion, the positive benefits/risk ratio of alfuzosin allows it to be classified as a uroselective α_1-blocker which provides a safe and effective contribution to the management of symptomatic BPH.

References

1 Barry MJ, Boyle P, Garraway M, Fang-Liu G, Guess HA, O'Leary P, Oishi R, Tsukamoto T: Epidemiology and natural history of BPH, in Cockett AT, Aso Y, Chatelain C, Denis L, Griffiths K, Khoury S, Murphy G (eds): Proc 2nd International Consultation on Benign Prostatic Hyperplasia (BPH). Jersey, Scientific Communications International, 1993, vol 2, pp 17–34.

2 Caine M, Pfau A, Pelberg S: The use of alpha-adrenergic blockers in benign prostatic obstruction. Br J Urol 1976;48:255–263.

3 Monda JM, Oesterling JE: Medical treatment of benign prostatic hyperplasia: 5α-Reductase inhibitors and α-adrenergic antagonists. Mayo Clin Proc 1993;68:670–679.

4 Andersson KE: Uroselectivity; in Cockett AT, Khoury S, Aso Y, Chatelain C, Denis L, Griffiths K, Murphy G (eds): Proc 3rd International Consultation on Benign Prostatic Hyperplasia (BPH). Jersey, Scientific Communications International, 1995, vol 3, pp 541–542.

5 Caine M: The present role of alpha-adrenergic blockers in the treatment of benign prostatic hypertrophy. J Urol 1986;136:1–4.

6 Shapiro E, Hartanto V, Lepor H: Anti-desmin vs. anti-actin for quantifying the area density of prostate smooth muscle. Prostate 1992;20: 259–267.

7 Furuya S, Kumamoto Y, Yokoyama E, Tsukamotot T, Izumi T, Abiko Y: Alpha-adrenergic activity and urethral pressure in prostatic zone in benign prostatic hypertrophy. J Urol 1982; 128:836–839.

8 Lepor H: Nonoperative management of benign prostatic hyperplasia. J Urol 1989;141:1283–1289.

9 Eri LM, Tveter KJ: α-Blockade in the treatment of symptomatic benign prostatic hyperplasia. J Urol 1995;154:923–934.

10 Jardin A, Bensadoun H, Delauche-Cavallier MC, Attali P, the BPH-ALF Group: Alfuzosin for treatment of benign prostatic hypertrophy. Lancet 1991;337:1457–1461.

11 Jardin A, Bensadoun H, Delauche-Cavallier MC, Attali P, the BPH-ALF Group: Long-term treatment of benign prostatic hyperplasia with alfuzosin: A 12–18 month assessment. Br J Urol 1993;72:615–620.

12 Jardin A, Bensadoun H, Delauche-Cavallier MC, Stalla-Bourdillon A, Attali P, the BPH-ALF Group: Long-term treatment of benign prostatic hyperplasia with alfuzosin: A 24–30 month survey. Br J Urol 1994;74:579–584.

13 Lukacs B, Leplège A, Thibault P, Jardin A: Prospective study in men with clinical benign prostatic hyperplasia treated with alfuzosin by general practitioners: 1-year results. Urology 1996; 48:731–740.

14 Lukacs B, Comet D, Doublet D, Gattegno B, Thibault P: Two-year assessment of long-term Health Related Quality of Life (HRQL) of 4591 patients suffering from benign prostatic hypertrophy (BPH) treated with a uroselective α_1-blocker, alfuzosin (abstract 1053). J Urol 1996;155(suppl)574A.

15 Teillac P, Delauche-Cavallier MC, Attali P, the DUALF Group: Urinary flow rates in patients with benign prostatic hypertrophy following treatment with alfuzosin. Br J Urol 1992;70:58–64.
16 Costa P, Geffriaud C, Delauche MC, Velut V, Proffit O, Bennaoum K, Bressolle F: Effect of a single dose of alfuzosin SR on flow rate in elderly patients with symptomatic benign prostatic hyperplasia (BPH) (abstract 45). Proc XIth Congr of the European Association of Urology, Berlin, 1994.
17 Greenberg RN: Overview of patients' compliance with medication dosing: A literature review. Clin Ther 1984;6:592–599.
18 Buzelin JM, Roth S, Geffriaud-Ricouard C, Delauche-Cavallier MC, the ALGEBI Study Group: Efficacy and safety of sustained-release alfuzosin 5 mg in patients with benign prostatic hyperplasia. Eur Urol 1997;31:190–198.
19 Buzelin JM, Herbert M, Blondin P, the PRAZALF Group: Alpha-blocking treatment with alfuzosin in symptomatic benign prostatic hyperplasia: Comparative study with prazosin. Br J Urol 1993;72:922–927.
20 Buzelin JM, Fonteyne E, Kontturi M, Witjes WPJ, Khan A for the European Tamsulosin Study Group. Comparison of tamsulosin with alfuzosin in the treatment of patients with lower urinary tract symptoms suggestive of bladder outlet obstructing (symptomatic benign prostatic hyperplasia). Br J Urol 1997;80:597–605.
21 Gillenwater JY, Conn RL, Chrysant SG, Roy J, Gaffney M, Ice K, Dias N, Multicenter Study Group: Doxazosin for the treatment of benign prostatic hyperplasia in patients with mild to moderate essential hypertension: A double-blind, placebo-controlled, dose-response multicenter study. J Urol 1995;154:110–115.
22 Roehrborn CG, Oesterling JE, Auerbach S, Kaplan SA, Lloyd K, Milam D, Padley R, HYCAT Investigator Group: Effectiveness and safety of terazosin versus placebo in the treatment of men with symptomatic benign prostatic hyperplasia in the HYCAT study. Urology 1996;47:169–178.
23 Berry SJ, Coffey DS, Walsh PC, Ewing L: The development of human benign prostatic hypertrophy with age. J Urol 1984;132:474–479.
24 Garraway WM, Collins GN, Lee RJ: High prevalence of benign prostatic hypertrophy in the community. Lancet 1991;338:469–471.
25 Lepor H, Williford WO, Barry MJ, Brawer MK, Dixon CM, Gormley G, Haakenson C, Machi M, Narayan P, Padley RJ for the Veterans Affairs Cooperative Studies Benign Prostatic Hyperplasia Study Group: The efficacy of terazosin, finasteride, or both in benign prostatic hypertrophy. New Engl J Med 1996;335:533–539.
26 Roehrborn CG, Siegel RL: Safety and efficacy of doxazosin in benign prostatic hyperplasia: A pooled analysis of three double-blind, placebo-controlled studies. Urology 1996;48:406–415.
27 Fawzy A, Braun K, Lewis GP, Gaffney M, Ice K, Dias N for the Multicenter Study Group: Doxazosin in the treatment of benign prostatic hyperplasia in normotensive patients: A multicenter study. J Urol 1995;154:105–109.
28 Graham RM, Thornell IR, Gain JM, Bagnoli C, Oates HF, Stokes GS: Prazosin: The first dose phenomenon. Br Med J 1976;2:1293–1294.
29 Takenaka T, Fujikura T, Honda K, Asano M, Niigata K: Discovery and development of tamsulosin hydrochloride, a new α_1-adrenoceptor antagonist. Yakugaku Zasshi 1995;115:773–789.
30 Myers MC, Kearns PM, Kennedy DS, Fischer RH: Postural hypotension and diuretic therapy in the elderly. Can Med Assoc J 1974;119:581–584.
31 Lipstiz LA: Orthostatic hypotension in the elderly. N Engl J Med 1989;321:952–956.
32 Lefèvre-Borg F, Lechaire J, O'Connor S: In vivo uroselectivity of alfuzosin compared to prazosin and terazosin (abstract 84). Br J Pharmacol 1992;106(suppl).
33 Martin DJ, Jammes D, Angel I: Effects of alfuzosin on urethral and blood pressures in conscious male rats. Life Sci 1995;57:PL387–391.
34 Martin D, Luel P, Guillot E, Coste A, Jammes D, Angel I: Comparative α_1-adrenoceptor subtype selectivity and functional uroselectivity of α_1-adrenoceptor antagonists. J Pharmacol Exp Ther 1997;282:228–235.
35 Rouquier L, Claustre Y, Benavides J: Alpha$_1$-adrenoceptor antagonists differentially control serotonin release in the hippocampus and striatum: A microdialysis study. Eur J Pharmacol 1994;261:59–64.
36 Scott MG, Deering AH, McMahon MT, Harron DWG, Shanks RG: Haemodynamic and pharmacokinetic evaluation of alfuzosin in man. A dose-ranging study and comparison with prazosin. Eur Clin Pharmacol 1989;37:53–58.
37 Buzelin JM, Delauche-Cavallier MC, Roth S, Geffriaud-Ricouard C, Santoni JP. Clinical uroselectivity: Evidence from patients treated with SR alfuzosin for symptomatic benign prostatic obstruction. Br J Urol 1997;79:898–906.
38 Lukacs B, Blondin P, McCarthy C, Du Boys B, Grippon P, Lassale C: Safety profile of 3 months' therapy with alfuzosin in 13,389 patients suffering from benign prostatic hypertrophy. Eur Urol 1996;29:29–35.
39 Stephenson TP, Jensen RD, PRANALF Group: A placebo-controlled study of the efficacy and tolerability of alfuzosin and prazosin for the treatment of benign prostatic hypertrophy (BPH) (abstract 48). Proc XIth Congr of the European Association of Urology, Berlin, 1994.
40 Delmas V, Coulange C, Caille P, Geffriaud C, Proffit O, Delauche-Cavallier MC: A placebo-controlled double-blind study of sustained release alfuzosin in benign prostatic hyperplasia (abstract 47). Proc XIth Congr of the European Association of Urology, Berlin, 1994.
41 Lowe FC: Safety assessment of terazosin in the treatment of patients with symptomatic benign prostatic hyperplasia: A combined analysis. Urology 1994;44:46–51.
42 Janknegt RA, Chapple CR for the Doxazosin Study Groups: Efficacy and safety of the α_1-blocker doxazosin in the treatment of benign prostatic hyperplasia. Analysis of 5 studies. Eur Urol 1993;24:319–326.
43 Abrams P, Schulman CC, Vaage S, European Tamsulosin Study Group: Tamsulosin, a selective α_{1C}-adrenoceptor antagonist: A randomized, controlled trial in patients with benign prostatic obstruction (symptomatic BPH). Br J Urol 1995;76:325–336.

European
Urology

Eur Urol 1998;33(suppl 2):28–33

B. Lukacs [a]
J.C. Grange [b]
C. McCarthy [b]
D. Comet [c]
BPH Group in General Practice

[a] Urology Department, Hospital Tenon, Paris,
[b] Laboratoires Synthélabo, Meudon,
[c] Département Biostatistique, Axonal, Nanterre, France

Clinical Uroselectivity: A 3-Year Follow-Up in General Practice

Key Words
BPH
Alfuzosin
Effectiveness
General practice
3-Year follow-up

Abstract
The objectives of this open-labeled study were to assess the clinical uroselectivity of alfuzosin in a long-term follow-up study in general practice. A total of 3,228 patients with clinical benign prostatic hyperplasia (BPH) from 812 centers were included in a prospective 3-year open-labeled study and treated with alfuzosin (immediate-release formulation) at the recommended dosage. Symptom score (Boyarsky, modified) and a 20-item BPH-specific health related quality of life (HRQL) score (Urolife™ BPH QoL 20), which included three questions on sexuality, were self-administered at baseline, 3, 6, 12, 18, 24, 30 and 36 months. Symptom score was significantly reduced by 54% at 3 months and this reduction was maintained up to 36 months; the HRQL score was significantly improved by 45.4% at 12 months and this improvement was also maintained up to 36 months. Alfuzosin was well tolerated: the quantitative and qualitative distribution of adverse events (AEs) was similar to that previously observed in placebo-controlled studies. 4.2% of the patients dropped out due to AEs. This study confirms the long-term safety profile of alfuzosin in general practice and highlights the need to measure HRQL in the context of clinical uroselectivity.

Introduction

In benign prostatic hyperplasia (BPH), α_1-blocker clinical uroselectivity can be defined as the desired effects on obstruction and lower urinary tract symptoms (LUTS) related to adverse events (AEs) [1]. Randomized, double-blind, placebo-controlled studies have consistently demonstrated the efficacy and safety of α_1-blockers for the treatment of BPH [2]. In particular, alfuzosin has been proven to have a good benefit/risk ratio [3, 4] and relatively high clinical uroselectivity [5]. Such efficacy studies, however, are not necessarily appropriate for informed decision making by primary-care practitioners [6]. The studies have inherent limitations in that a highly selected patient population is recruited. In addition, they generally assess symptoms and classical measurements, such as uroflow and residual urine, but they do not take into account the impact of symptoms on individual patients [7]. Another limitation is that patient's preferences for therapy are not taken into account. To address these limitations a long-term, open-labeled study was conducted involving a representative population of patients with

KARGER
Fax + 41 61 306 12 34
E-Mail karger@karger.ch
www.karger.com

0302–2838/98/0338–0028$15.00/0

This article is also accessible online at:
http://BioMedNet.com/karger

Dr. B. Lukacs
Hôpital Tenon
4, rue de la Chine
F–75020 Paris (France)
Tel. +33 1 40 30 70 00, Fax +33 1 40 30 61 52

clinical BPH and treated as closely as possible to routine practice in the community. The study measured the effectiveness of treatment with regard to symptoms and their impact on patient's perceived health status. As BPH can be considered as a quality of life (QoL) disease [8], measures of symptoms and BPH health status can be expected to be the most accurate and sensitive assessments of treatment effectiveness from the patient's perspective [9]. A self-administered, disease-specific health-related quantity of life (HRQL) questionnaire was developed, as recommended by the Third International Consultation on BPH [10]. This comprised 20 visual-analogue scale items and examined four dimensions including patient's perceived sexual drive assessment (Urolife™ BPH QoL 20) [11]. The basic requirements of HRQL measurements were: multidimensional (to give a picture of the overall health status of the patient); reliable (test-retest reliability); valid (is the questionnaire measuring what it intended to measure); sensitive to change (response to treatment); appropriate (specific to the clinical condition under study); and practical (in the conditions of routine practice) [12]. Finally, it could be stated that α_1-blocker clinical uroselectivity assessment should primarily evaluate the benefit/risk ratio; but the safety profile must be completed by the construct and the study of a large patient data base including nonselected patients such as middle-aged, elderly patients and patients taking multiple medication. So, effectiveness studies can be defined as how the drug works in the community settings and how the patient perceives his treatment.

Methods

Patients aged less than 85 years with clinical BPH were enrolled in the study after informed consent. Concomitant medication with another α_1-blocker was prohibited, but use of plant extracts was allowed if such treatment was not initiated or modified during the trial. Patients were excluded if they had urological symptoms due to another urinary tract disorder, had previously undergone prostate surgery, or were scheduled for surgery within the next 3 months.

Alfuzosin was administered at standard dosage, in accordance with French data recommendations. The dosage regimen was 2.5 mg t.i.d. (7.5 mg/day) orally for 36 months. Symptoms were measured using a standardized self-administered BPH symptom questionnaire (including the nine items of the Boyarsky score [13] and one additional item 'straining to void') completed at the primary-care practitioner's office at baseline and at 1, 3, 6, 12, 18, 24, 30 and 36 months. Symptoms were classified as storage (irritative) (day-time frequency, nocturia, urgency) or voiding (obstructive) (quality of urine stream, feeling of incomplete voiding, straining to urinate, intermittency) symptoms. Each question scored on a scale from 0–40 and patients were stratified according to symptom severity: mild symptoms (0–13), moderate symptoms (14–26) and severe symptoms (27–40).

Table 1. BPH-specific HRQL questionnaire (QoL 20)

Physical/functional dimension	
	q2 – Stopping to urinate
	q3 – Quality of sleep
	q4 – Appetite
	q5 – Sexual desire
	q9 – Urgent micturition
	q11 – Erection
Social status dimension	
	q1 – Social activities
	q8 – Familial activities
	q10 – Leisure pursuits
	q14 – Adapting to situations
	q17 – Satisfaction with sex-life
	q20 – Relations with others
Mental health status dimension	
	q6 – Memory
	q7 – Fatigue
	q12 – Concentration
	q13 – Energy, vitality
	q15 – Mood
	q18 – Anxiety
Overall QoL	
	q16 – Love of life
	q19 – Satisfaction with current life

HRQL was measured using a validated disease-specific HRQL questionnaire (Urolife BPH QoL 20), which was self-administered at the primary-care practitioner's office at baseline and 3, 6, 12, 18, 24, 30 and 36 months. This specific questionnaire consisted of 20 questions (table 1) scored on 10-cm visual-analogue scales (VAS), the minimum and maximum scores for each question were 0 and 10, respectively. The global HRQL score was calculated by summing the 18 VAS scores for the three dimensions physical/functional (six questions), social life (six questions) and mental health (six questions), and the two VAS scores for the overall (QoL) dimension (two questions). The sum of the scores for each dimension gave three corresponding subscores (0–60), and an overall QoL subscore (0–200) was calculated by combining the three subscores and those of the two general questions. Three of the questions included the patient's perceived sexual life status: two were from the physical/functional subscore (sexual desire, quality of erection) and one from the social life subscore (satisfaction with sexual life). These were analysed separately by constructing a sexuality subscore (0–30).

Safety was assessed by gathering reports of AEs in an open mode and by blood pressure and heart rate measurements at each visit.

Demographic characteristics and safety were analysed on an intent-to-treat basis. Analysis for possible efficacy-related factors was carried out by simple regression, χ^2 test, or an analysis of variance (Anova), depending on the type of data. All analyses were two-tailed

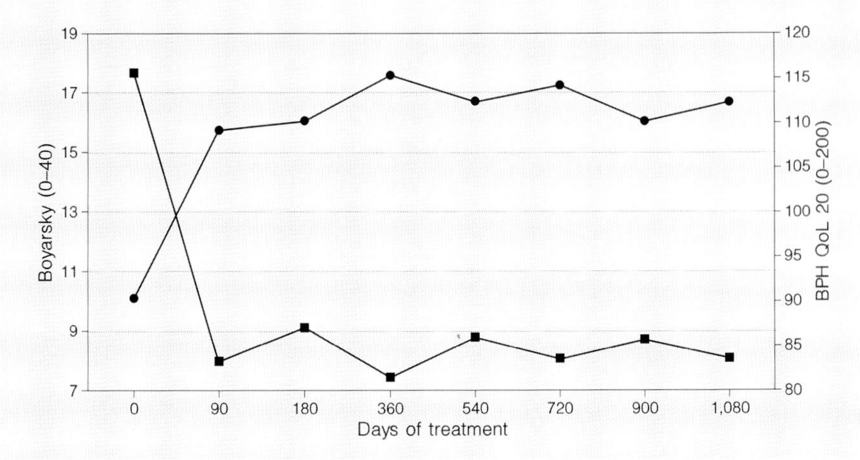

Fig. 1. Changes in Boyarsky symptom (■) and HRQL Urolife BPH QL20 (●) scores up to 3 years.

with a level of 5%. Results were expressed as mean (± SEM). Data changes were analysed by: (a) measurement of absolute variation (last value-baseline value); (b) measurement of relative variation ([last value – baseline value]/ baseline value), and (c) measurement of magnitude of therapeutic effect or Effect Size Index (ESI) ([last value – baseline value]/baseline value standard deviation). For discrete variables, analysis was carried out using the χ^2 test, with regrouping if necessary, and Fisher's exact test. For continuous variables, Pearson's linear regression was performed using the least-squares rule, completed if necessary by stepwise regression, and Anova for repeated measures, for the parameters analysed at the various study periods. A multivariate analysis (multiple correspondence analysis [MCA]) was also used to detect patient profiles.

Analyses were performed using SAS software 6.1.0. (SAS Institute, Cary, NC, USA).

Results

Patients' Characteristics

A total of 3,228 patients (mean age: 66.9 ± 0.1) were enrolled by 812 French primary-care practitioners; 2,579 patients (79.9%) completed the 3-year study. Of the patients enrolled, 649 (20.1%) withdrew from the study for the following reasons: death (n = 245; 7.6%), AE (135; 4.2%), lost to follow-up (55; 1.7%), lack of efficacy (60; 1.8%), study withdrawal for personal reason (26; 0.8%), concomitant disease (23; 0.7%), or other reason (105; 3.3%). One hundred and twenty patients (3.7%) were operated on and 9 patients (0.3%) experienced acute urinary retention. The only factor correlated with withdrawal was the lack of QoL improvement (ESI): 0.10 vs. 0.68 ($p < 0.0001$] for patients who withdrew (deaths excluded) and for patients who completed the study, respectively. Patients who underwent surgery during the study experienced less symptom improvement than those not operated on (ESI: 0.25 vs 1.29; $p < 0.0001$).

A total of 1,224 patients (39.0%) were aged less than 65 years, 929 (29.6%) were aged 65–70 years, and 982 patients (31.3%) were aged over 70 years. The mean duration of the disease at baseline was 37.3 ± 0.62 months. Mean prostate volume measured in 2,503 patients was 50.2 ± 0.6. Ultrasonography was performed on 2,748 patients with a residual urine measured in 1,806 patients (65.7%); 978 patients showed a residual urine of more than 30 ml (mean 101.2 ± 2.9 ml). Comorbidity was present in 2,272 patients (70.4%) and 2,233 (69.2%) were treated with at least one concomitant therapy: 1,129 received antihypertensive treatment or nitrate derivatives; 318, an ACE inhibitor; 266, a calcium antagonist; 187, a diuretic; 145, a β-blocker; 141, a nitrate derivative; and 82, other treatments. According to the Boyarsky modified score, the majority of patients reported moderate symptoms (1998; 63.5%) versus patients reporting mild and severe symptoms: 782 (24.8%) and 368 (11.7%), respectively. Mean scores (± SEM) for nocturia and daytime frequency were 3.25 ± 0.02 and 7.60 ± 0.04, respectively, HRQL score was negatively correlated with age ($r = -0.26$, $p < 0.0001$). Symptom severity (categorizing in mild/moderate/severe classes) and impaired QoL were strongly negatively correlated ($r = -0.46$, $p < 0.0001$]. Patient's perceived sexual life subscore was negatively correlated with age ($r = -0.34$, $p < 0.0001$) and with symptom severity ($r = -0.46$, $p = 0.0001$).

Effect of Treatment

Symptom Score (Boyarsky, Modified). Baseline Boyarsky modified symptom score (17.6 ± 0.1) was sig-

Table 2. Baseline, 3-year values, absolute and percentage improvements in Boyarsky symptom score by symptom severity

		Score, day 0 (0–40)	Score, day 1,080 (0–40)	Mean change	Mean change, %		ESI day 1,080
					of baseline	of 40	
All patients	n	3,148	2,437	2,391	2,389	2,391	2,391
		17.64 (0.12)	8.02 (0.10)	9.65 (0.16)	48.42 (0.77)	24.13 (0.40)	1.39 (0.02)
Mild symptoms	n	782	584	584	582	584	584
		9.44 (0.08)	6.78 (0.18)	2.60 (0.19)	24.46 (2.16)	6.50 (0.47)	0.37 (0.03)
Moderate symptoms	n	1,998	1,528	1,528	1,528	1,528	1,528
		18.47 (0.09)	8.26 (0.12)	10.19 (0.15)	53.60 (0.72)	24.48 (0.38)	1.46 (0.02)
Severe symptoms	n	368	279	279	279	279	279
		30.56 (0.16)	9.05 (0.34)	21.46 (0.39)	70.03 (1.14)	53.66 (0.97)	3.08 (0.06)

Figures in parentheses represent standard error of the mean. ESI = Mean change divided by the standard deviation of the baseline score. $p < 0.0001$ for comparisons between severity classes.

nificantly reduced ($p = 0.0001$) at 3, 6, 12, 18, 24 and 36 months (fig. 1). The onset of maximum symptom reduction occurred at the first measurement after 3 months of treatment (–9.87 ± 0.11; –54.0%) and was maintained up to 3 years (–9.65 ± 0.16; –48.4%). Table 2 shows the variations of symptom score according to baseline symptom severity expressed as absolute improvement, percentage improvement (of baseline and of scale range) and magnitude of effect (ESI), (the comparisons between severity classes were all significant: $p < 0.0001$). Storage (range 0–12) and voiding scores (range 0–16) were significantly reduced ($p = 0.0001$) from baseline at 36 months: –53.7% and –38.3%, respectively. In patients who completed both initial and 3-year symptom questionnaires, the 3-year symptom profile was improved compared to the baseline symptom profile: of the 1,528 patients reporting moderate symptoms at baseline, 1,295 (84.8%) were improved, 225 (14.7%) remained clinically stable, and 8 (0.5%) reported worsening of their symptoms; of the 279 patients reporting severe symptoms at baseline, 218 (78.1%) and 60 (21.6%) reported mild and moderate symptoms at 36 months, respectively, and 1 patient (0.4%) remained severely symptomatic after a 36-month treatment; of the 584 patients reporting mild symptoms at baseline, 43 (7.4%) reported worsening symptoms after treatment. After 36 months of treatment and according to the magnitude of effect (ESI), symptoms were improved (ESI >0.5) in 1,887 patients (78.9%), stabilized (0 < ESI ≤0.5) in 432 patients (18.1%) and worsened (ESI < 0.5] in 72 patients (3.0%).

HRQL score (Urolife™ BPH QoL 20). Baseline HRQL score (90.4 ± 6) was significantly ($p < 0.0001$) improved at 3, 6, 12, 18, 24, 30 and 36 months (fig. 1). Maximum HRQL improvement occurred at 12 months (+25.11 ± 0.77; +45.4%) and was maintained up to 3 years (+21.41 ± 0.9; +43.4%). Improvement in physical/functional dimension was greater (ESI = 0.88) than in social dimension (ESI = 0.62), mental dimension (ESI = 0.45), and patient's perceived sexual dimension (ESI = 0.37). HRQL improvement was more strongly negatively correlated with baseline symptom severity than with age (table 3). Patient's perceived sexual life subscore improvement (ESI) was strongly negatively correlated with age and with initial symptom severity; however, according to ESI > 0.5 and age, it was significantly improved in patients reporting severe symptoms at baseline regardless of their age: 1.04, 1.06 and 0.67 in younger, middle-aged and older patients, respectively (table 3).

Safety

During the 3-year treatment, 655 AEs occurred in 413 patients (12.8%); 262 patients (8.1%) experienced severe AEs (comprising 245 deaths [7.6%]), 151 patients (4.7%) presented 295 nonsevere AEs. The main AEs (deaths excepted) were: vertigo (n = 43, 1.3%), dizziness (27, 0.8%), nausea (24, 0.7%), malaise (27, 0.7%), headache (20, 0.6%), abdominal pain (16, 0.5%), hypotension (13, 0.4%) and palpitation (11, 0.3%). There were no clinically significant changes in systolic and diastolic blood pressure or heart rate between baseline and 3 years.

Table 3. Magnitudes of effects (ESI) for symptoms and HRQL after a 36-month treatment with alfuzosin according to age and baseline symptom severity

	All patients	Symptom severity			p (intra class)
		mild	moderate	severe	
Age < 65 year					
Symptoms	1.39	0.49	1.57	3.19	0.0001
HRQL	0.72	0.30	0.78	1.67	0.0001
Sexual drive	0.38	0.14	0.41	1.04	0.0001
65 ≤ age ≤ 70 years					
Symptoms	1.40	0.28	1.47	3.28	0.0001
HRQL	0.71	0.06	0.76	1.61	0.0001
Sexual drive	0.43	–0.04	0.48	1.06	0.0001
Age > 70 years					
Symptoms	1.40	0.17	1.32	2.89	0.0001
HRQL	0.59	0.07	0.61	0.91	0.0001
Sexual drive	0.30	–0.06	0.28	0.67	0.0001
p (intra age)					
Symptoms	0.88	0.0001	0.0003	0.02	
HRQL	0.13	0.09	0.149	0.0004	
Sexual drive	0.05	0.23	0.01	0.045	

Discussion

α_1-Blocker clinical uroselectivity can be considered as the balance between efficacy and safety or, more precisely, as the desired effects on obstruction and LUTS related to adverse effects. In disease areas such as BPH, the positive benefit/risk ratio observed in placebo-controlled randomized trials should be confirmed in large cohort studies in general practice. The common and chronic condition of BPH supposes that a large population of nonselected BPH patients, such as middle-aged, sexually active, and the elderly with a high rate of comorbidity, are likely to be treated in such studies. It is then necessary to assess how their disease-specific health status is affected by the treatment. Long-term effectiveness studies are relevant in the perspective of individual treatment decisions and can provide information on how to manage such a chronic disease and how to inform patients about their condition. The measurement of clinical uroselectivity must include symptom score, safety profile and health status assessment. According to the Food and Drug Administration, a multidimensional BPH-specific HRQL questionnaire is more appropriate than a single disease-specific question to capture the impact of symptoms on the health status of BPH patients at baseline and more sensitive to changes during the course of treatment [14].

Patients enrolled in this trial were those seeking medical therapy for relief of their LUTS. It was not possible to include a control group because patients were unlikely to agree to undergo watchful waiting for a period of 36 months. No group control was included in the present study conducted in the community practice setting for 3 years. Similarly, no urodynamic assessment was performed: the patients were included whatever their degree of bladder outlet obstruction; subsequent studies have shown that initial bladder outlet obstruction severity did not influence symptom score reduction due to surgery [15] or α_1-blocker therapy [16].

The overall results of the study indicate a strong negative correlation between symptom score reduction (–48.4%) and HRQL improvement (+43.4%) after a 3-year treatment (fig. 1). This would suggest that HRQL measurement is unnecessary except that individual patient characteristics such as age, baseline symptom severity or patient's perceived sexual drive dimension, appear to be important factors. At baseline it was confirmed that HRQL score and patient's perceived sexual drive dimension were negatively correlated with age and symptom severity. During the course of treament, the onset of maximum symptom score reduction and maximum HRQL improvement occurred at 3 and 12 months, respectively. It was also confirmed that physical/functional dimension was more improved than social life status and mental dimensions [17] which contrasts with the findings of Fowler et al. [18] and of Doll et al. [19]. Storage symptom score was significantly more reduced than voiding symptom score which is consistent with the fact that storage symptoms were perceived by the patients as the most bothersome [20] and the most correlated with QoL responses [21]. Patient's perceived sexual drive was significantly improved in the patients reporting the most severe symptoms at baseline regardless of their age. It should be noted that clinical sexual score assessment [22] is different from the BPH patient's perception of his sexual status. In BPH, the majority of patients do not complain about sexual function but are concerned about treatments which might interfere with their sexual life status.

The present study confirms the good safety profile of alfuzosin: the quantitative and qualitative distribution of AEs was similar to that previously observed in placebo-controlled studies [3, 4]. Deaths during this 3-year study (245; 7.6%), were consistent with the rate expected in a similar population of men (0.8% per 90 days) (7). The incidence of withdrawals from the study due to AEs was low (4.2%) as compared to the figure of 19% observed in a 42-month open trial conducted with terazosin (19%) [23].

The present data highlight the necessity of conducting effectiveness studies complementary to efficacy studies. HRQL assessment in BPH patients is necessary in order to evaluate the impact of symptoms on the patient's health status. It explores dimensions different from symptom score assessment and must include a sexual status element. Clinical uroselectivity assessment addresses benefit/risk ratio, long-term safety profile in the community and the patient's treatment preferences. The positive benefit/risk ratio of alfuzosin allows it to be classified as a uroselective α_1-blocker which provides a beneficial contribution to the management of symptomatic BPH.

References

1 Andersson KE, Lepor H, Wyllie MG: Prostatic α_1-adrenoreceptors and uroselectivity. Prostate 1997;30:202–215.

2 Eri LM, Tveter KJ: α-Blockade in the treatment of symptomatic benign prostatic hyperplasia. J Urol 1995;154:923–934.

3 Jardin A, Bensaddoun H, Delauche-Cavalier MC, Attali P, and the BPH-ALF Group: Alfuzosin for treatment of benign prostatic hypertrophy. Lancet 1991;337:1457–1461.

4 Buzelin JM, Roth S, Geffriaud-Ricouard C, Delauche-Cavallier MC and the Algebi study group: Efficacy and safety of sustained-release alfuzosin 5 mg in patients with benign prostatic hyperplasia. Eur Urol 1997;31:190–198.

5 Buzelin JM, Delauche-Cavallier MC, Roth S, Geffriaud-Ricouard C, Santoni JP: Clinical uroselectivity: Evidence from patients treated with slow-release alfuzosin for symptomatic benign prostatic obstruction. Br J Urol 1997; 79:898–906.

6 Iezzoni LI: Risk adjustment for medical outcome studies; in Grady ML, Schwartz HA (eds): Medical Effectiveness Research Data Methods. Rockville, Agency for Health Care Policy and Research, 1992, pp 83–97.

7 Guess HA, Chute CG, Garraway WM, Girman CJ, Panser LA, Lee RJ, Jacobsen SJ, McKelvie GB, Oesterling JE, Lieber MM: Similar levels of urological symptoms have similar impact on Scottish and American men – although Scots report less symptoms. J Urol 1993;150:1701–1705.

8 Mc Connel JD, Barry MJ, Bruskewitz RC, Bueschen AJ, Denton SE Holtgrewe HL, Lange JL, McClennan BL, Mebust WK, Reilly NJ, Roberts RG, Sacks SA, Wasson JH: Benign prostatic hyperplasia: Diagnosis and treatment. Clinical Practice Guideline, No 8. AHCPR Publication No. 94–0582. Rockville, Agency for Health Care Policy and Research, 1994, p 225.

9 Barry MJ, Fowler FJ, O'Leary M, Bruskewitz RC, Holtgrewe HL, Mebust WK: Measuring disease-specific health status in men with benign prostatic hyperplasia. Med Care 1995;33 (suppl):AS145–155.

10 Mebust WK, Donovan J, Bosch R, Okada K, O'Leary M, Batista J, Boyle P, Villers A, Ackermann R, Hoke G, Lukacs B, Mortensen S: Symptoms evaluation, quality of life and sexuality; in Cockett ATK, Khoury S, Aso Y, Chatelain C, Denis L, Griffiths K, et al (eds): Proceedings of the Third International Consultation on Benign Prostatic Hyperpasia (BPH). Jersey, Scientific Communications International, 1996, pp 257–261.

11 Lukacs B, Leplege A, Mc Carthy C, Comet D: Construction and validation of a BPH specific health related quality of life scale (with special attention to sexuality), for medical outcome research studies; in Cockett ATK, Khoury S, Aso Y et al (eds): Proceedings of the Second International Consultation on Benign Prostatic Hyperplasia (BPH). Jersey, Scientific Communications International, 1994, pp 139–143.

12 Fitzpatrick R, Fletcher A, Gore S, Jones D, Spiegelhalter D, Cox D: Quality of life measures in health care. I. Applications and issues in assessment. Br Med J 1992;305:1074–1077.

13 Boyarsky S, Jones G, Paulson DF, Prout GR: A new look at bladder neck obstruction by the Food and Drug Administration regulators: Guidelines for investigation of benign prostatic hypertrophy. Trans Am Assoc Genito-Urin Surg 1977;68:29–32.

14 Comparing treatments: safety, effectiveness, and cost-effectiveness. March 23rd/24th Workshop. FDA, Division of drug marketing, advertising and promotion (DDMAC). Principles for the review of pharmacoeconomic promotion. Script No 2013, April 4th, 1995.

15 Van Mastrigt R, Rollema HJ: The prognostic value of bladder contractility in transurethral resection of the prostate. J Urol 1992;148: 1856–1860.

16 Lepor H, Nieder A, Feser J, O'Connell C, Dixon C: Effect of terazosin on prostatism in men with normal and abnormal peak urinary flow rates. Urology 1997;49:476–480.

17 Lukacs B, Leplage A, Thibault P, Jardin A: Prospective study of men with clinical benign prostatic hyperplasia treated with alfuzosin by general practitioners: 1-year results. Urology 1996; 48:731–740.

18 Fowler FJ, Wennberg JE, Timothy RP, Barry MJ, Mulley AG, Hanley D: Symptom status and quality of life following prostatectomy. J Am Med Assoc 1988;259:3018–3022.

19 Doll HA, Black NA, Flood AB, McPherson K, Williams GB, Smith JC: Differences in outcome of TURP for benign prostatic hypertrophy between three diagnostic categories. Br J Urol 1993;72:322–330.

20 Jolleys JV, Donovan JL, Nanchahal K, Peters TJ, Abrams P: Urinary symptoms in the community: How bothersome are they? Br J Urol 1994;74:551–555.

21 The Department of Veterans Affairs Cooperative Study of transurethral resection for benign prostatic hyperplasia. A comparison of quality of life with patient reported symptoms and objective findings in men with benign prostatic hyperplasia. J Urol 1993;150:1696–1700.

22 O'Leary MP, Fowler FJ, Lenderking WR, Barber B, Sagnier PP, Guess HA, Barry M: A brief male sexual function inventory for urology. Urology 1995;46:697–706.

23 Lepor H: Long-term efficacy and safety of terazosin in patients with benign prostatic hyperplasia. Urology 1995;45:406–413.

European
Urology

Roger S. Kirby

Concluding Remarks

With the greying of the baby boomers, prostatic diseases particularly benign prostatic hyperplasia (BPH), have received unparalleled attention. BPH is now established as an important public health problem affecting many millions of men worldwide. In spite of the gradual onset of lower urinary tract symptoms (LUTS), BPH is not uncommonly associated with a reduced quality of life, and it is this that eventually drives patients to seek advice from urologists about the various treatment options available.

Until recently, surgery with transurethral prostatectomy (TURP) has been the first-line therapy for symptomatic BPH. Heightened awareness, however, among the general public and primary-care practitioners alike has led to earlier presentation of patients. Those with less severe symptoms and only modest obstruction are obvious candidates for medical rather than surgical therapy. These men are often reluctant to submit themselves to surgery without at least a trial of medical treatment in the first instance. In fact, the more severe the symptoms the greater the effect produced by medical therapy.

But which pharmacological agent should the attending physician select to commence therapy? Clearly what the patient wants is a compound with maximum efficacy and only minimal side effects. It is here that the concept of 'uroselectivity' translates into actual clinical value. The optimum BPH therapy should reduce LUTS, enhance uroflow and improve quality of life at a cost of side effects not greatly exceeding those of placebo. In this respect, the newer α-blockers, such as alfuzosin, seem to have an advantage over older agents.

Nobody knows precisely what the future holds, but the use of medical therapy for BPH as first-line treatment seems certain to increase. As the new millenium dawns and the world's population ages, more and more men are likely to present with LUTS as a result of BPH. Consequently, an ever-increasing number of them seems likely to receive, in the short and longer term, uroselective agents such as alfuzosin which has been the subject of this excellent symposium.

KARGER
Fax + 41 61 306 12 34
E-Mail karger@karger.ch
www.karger.com

This article is also accessible online at:
http://BioMedNet.com/karger

European Association of Urology

MEMBERSHIP APPLICATION

Name: . . . .
(last) (first & middle) (title)

Date of birth: ... - ... -19..

Mailing address: . . . .

. . . .

Zip code/City: . . . .

Country: . . . .

Phone number: . . . . FAX number: . . . .

❑ Active membership ❑ Affiliated membership

❑ Corresponding membership

❑ Junior membership

Please mark with x the membership you are applying for.

Certification as Urologist

- Country: . . . .
- Date of certification: . . . .
- Authority which had delivered the certification: . . . .
  (please enclose copy)

Sponsor (Name of a *Active Member* of the EAU who supports your application)

. . . .

Certification as Urologist-in-Training

- Country: . . . .
- Date of starting the education as urologist in training: . . . .
- Statement of Chief of your department indicating that you are a urologist-in-training
  (please enclose copy)

Sponsor (Name of a Active Member of the EAU who supports your application)

. . . .

MEMBERSHIP CATEGORIES

Admission Regulations

Active membership
Active membership is open to all registered urologists in Europe.
The application has to be endorsed by one Active Member of the EAU. Active Members have the right to vote at the General Assembly.
Application is made directly to the EAU Central Office, accompanied by a certificate of registration as a urologist in the applicant's European country.

Junior membership
Junior membership is open to European urologists-in-training. The application has to be endorsed by one Active Member of the EAU. Junior Members have no right to vote at the General Assembly.
Application is made directly to the EAU Central Office accompanied by a letter from the Chief of his/her department indicating that he/she is a urologist-in-training.
Upon registration as a urologist, Junior members may apply to become Active Members

Senior membership
Senior membership is open to Active Members officially retired (at their own request)
Senior members have no right to vote at the General Assembly.
Senior members are exempted from any fees payable to the Association.

Corresponding membership
Corresponding membership is open to all registered non-European urologists. The application has to be endorsed by two Active Members of the EAU.
Corresponding Members have no right to vote at the General Assembly.
Application is made directly to the EAU Central Office, accompanied by a certificate of registration as a urologist in the applicant's own country or an endorsement by their national society.

Affiliate membership
Affiliate membership is open to all scientists or others who have contributed significantly to the specialty of urology. The application has to be endorsed by two Active members.
Application is made directly to the EAU Central Office accompanied with a curriculum vitae and other pertinent information as well as a signed document that they are not connected with any commercial or pharmaceutical company.

Honorary membership
Honorary membership may be awarded to scientists and others who have had an important influence on European urology. Their election will be recommended by the Board and must be approved by the General Assembly.

MEMBERSHIP FEES

Active members will have to pay NLG 250 per year (including subscription to European Urology).
Corresponding members will have to pay NLG 315 per year (including subscription to European Urology).
Junior members will have to pay NLG 150 per year (including subscription to European Urology).
Affiliated members will have to pay NLG 200 per year (including subscription to European Urology).

Please enclose payment with your membership application.

Methods of payments

Please make your bank transfer or cheque, in Dutch guilders only, payable to:

European Urological Foundation (EAU), account number: 22.59.17.726.
Bank relation: F. van Lanschot, bankers, Nijmegen, the Netherlands.

Credit cards: ❑ **American Express** ❑ **Visa**

card number: .... **expiry date:** ....

signature: ....

PLEASE RETURN THIS APPLICATION TO:

The EAU Office
P.O. Box 204
6600 AE Wijchen
the Netherlands

phone: +31-24-6452510
fax: +31-24-6450769